Easy P Recipes

Vegan, Gluten-Free, Oil-Free Cookbook for Lifelong Health

Helena Esquibel

HELENA ESQUIBEL

Easy Plant-Based Recipes

Table of Contents

INTRODUCTION 1

BREAKFAST 1

1. SMOKY, SAUCY BLACK-EYED PEAS 3
2. POTATO SALAD WITH AVOCADO AND DILL 5
3. MINESTRONE IN MINUTES 8
4. BROCOLLI SOUP 10
5. RED LENTIL DAL 12

BAKED AND STUFFED 14

6. TWICE-BAKED SWEET POTATOES 15
7. MILLET LOAF 17
8. SMOKY LITTLE DEVILS 19
9. MUSHROOM-BASIL AU GRATIN 21
10. EGGPLANT ROLLATINI 24
11. EGGPLANT CANNELLONI WITH BRAVO TOMATO SAUCE 27
12. SWEET POTATO, PEAR, AND BLUEBERRY FLATBREADS 30
13. KIWI-ORANGE FLATBREADS 32
14. VEGAN BUTTERNUT SQUASH LASAGNA ROLL-UPS 34
15. EASY BAKE BEAN 37
16. GREEK STUFFED PEPPERS 39
17. OVEN-BAKED CHICKPEA RATATOUILLE 41

VEGAN GRAIN RECIPIES 43

18. RED BEANS & QUINOA 44
19. WILD RICE, CABBAGE AND CHICKPEA PILAF 46
20. BURRITO BOWL 48
21. WHOLE GRAIN STUFFING WITH PECANS AND CURRANT 50
22. CURRIED MILLET CAKES WITH CREAMY RED PEPPER CORIANDER ... 52
23. BASIC POLENTA 54
24. BARLEY AND SWEET POTATO PILAF 55

SNACKS AND APPETIZERS 57

25. SPICY FRENCH FRIES 58
26. CHEESY" VEGGIE PIZZETTES 60
27. CRISPY BUFFALO CAULIFLOWER BITES 63
28. BANANA BLUEBERRY BARS 65

29.   Yamadillas.. 67

30.   Mexican 10-Layer Dip..................................... 69

PASTA & NOODLES 71

31.   Spaghetti with Roasted Tomatoes, Chickpeas, and Basil 72

32.   White Beans with Greens, Garlic and Tomato 74

33.   Rip's Pasta Primavera 76

34.   Roasted Tomato and Cannellini Bean Pasta........................ 77

35.   Mediterranean Vegetable Spaghetti 79

36.   Fettuccine with Grilled Asparagus, Peas, and Lemon 81

37.   Ponzu Noodle Salad 83

38.   Velvety Macaroni.. 85

39.   Pasta Primavera 87

40.   Thai Green Curry Rice................................. 90

DESSERTS 91

41.   Cranberry-Orange Biscotti 92

42.   Chocolate Chip Pumpkin Muffins................. 94

43.   Blackberry-Peach Cobbler........................... 96

44.   No-Bake Cranberry Pear Tart 99

45.   Indian Brown Rice Pudding (Kheer)............. 101

46.   Southern-Style Banana Pudding Parfaits 103

47.   Purple Sticky Rice Pudding 105

48.   Strawberry Clafouti Dessert 106

49.   Fruit-Topped Vanilla Cupcakes 108

50.   Sweet Potato Bites...................................... 111

51.   Cantaloupe-Cucumber Soup 112

52.   Chocolate Pistachio Mint and Strawberry Rose Bliss Balls 113

53.   Brownies 115

54.   Hidden Berry Dessert Squares..................... 117

55.   Cherry Soft-Serve Ice Cream....................... 119

56.   Fruit & Spice Cookies 120

INTRODUCTION

The plant-based diet is not so much of a diet as it is a lifestyle change. If you have been a vegetarian for most of your life, you are going to have to change how much you eat as well as your eating habits. However, for those that are switching from an omnivorous way of life to a plant-based lifestyle, it is going to be quite a challenge. Not only will you have to change the way you eat, what you eat, and how much you eat - you'll have to change your habits as well. You will have to change the way you shop, the way you cook, make better menu choices at restaurants, and make sure everyone knows of your lifestyle change. If you have your own family, you may find yourself having to cook two completely different dinners or adapting your plant-based one to fit theirs. There are always ways around certain food challenges, but the main thing is being forthright with your dietary changes to those closest to you. The reason so many diets fail is that they are either fad diets or people get fed up with them as they are too complicated. They also tend to rush headlong into a diet and go cold turkey. That is no way to approach a diet, let alone a complete lifestyle change. Choosing a plant-based diet to lose weight, for health reasons, or for a healthier lifestyle you need to start with the right approach towards the diet. With that said, the time and effort you put into transitioning to a plant-based diet will be worth it in terms of your health, as well as the health of the planet.

BREAKFAST

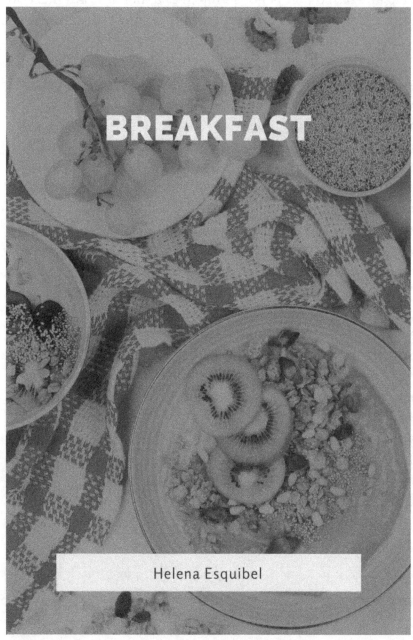

1.<u>SMOKY, SAUCY BLACK-EYED PEAS</u>

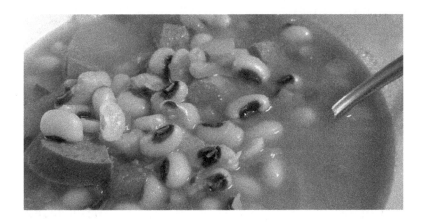

This hearty soup recipe is an excellent way to transform frozen black-eyed peas into a filling vegan meal. Add chopped fresh (or canned) tomatoes, bell pepper, and corn, and season with chipotle chili powder, paprika, cumin, and fresh cilantros

INGREDIENTS

- 1 cup chopped onion
- 1 cup chopped red bell pepper
- 2 cups frozen black-eyed peas
- 1 cup chopped ripe tomatoes with their juices
- 2 cups boiling water
- 1½ cups fresh or frozen corn
- ½ cup snipped fresh cilantro
- 2 teaspoons smoked paprika
- 1½ teaspoons agave syrup
- ½ teaspoon dried oregano, crushed
- ½ teaspoon ground chipotle chili pepper

- ¼ teaspoon ground cumin

- Sea salt, to taste

INSTRUCTIONS

- In a large saucepan, cook onion over medium heat for 7 to 8 minutes, stirring occasionally and adding water, 1 to 2 tablespoons at a time, as needed to prevent sticking. Add bell pepper; cook 5 minutes. Add frozen black-eyed peas and tomatoes with juices. Cook, covered, over medium-low heat 5 minutes.

- Stir in 2 cups boiling water, corn, cilantro, paprika, agave syrup, oregano, chipotle pepper, and cumin. Cook, partially covered, over medium-low heat 35 minutes. If necessary cook 10 to 15 minutes more or until black-eyed peas are tender. Season with salt. Sprinkle with addition

2. <u>POTATO SALAD WITH AVOCADO AND DILL</u>

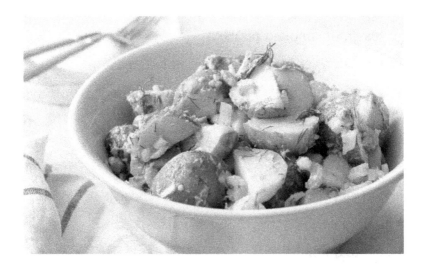

This hearty soup recipe is an excellent way to transform frozen black-eyed peas into a filling vegan meal. Add chopped fresh (or canned) tomatoes, bell pepper, and corn, and season with chipotle chili powder, paprika, cumin, and fresh cilantro.

When using whole foods, how do you make a creamy potato salad? It's that easy! Mash up a fresh ripe avocado and use it in place of the vegan mayo (an ingredient I do not use in my kitchen!) I like to season this recipe to give it a little extra kick, so it's a dish that can be enjoyed on its own or with a light soup or wrap. Prepare to taste the best whole-food potato salad you've ever had

INGREDIENTS

- 2 pounds small red potatoes
- 1 large avocado

- 2 teaspoons fresh lemon juice

- 1 tablespoon Dijon mustard

- ¼ teaspoon smoked paprika

- ½ teaspoon (or less) Herbamare or sea salt

- 1½ teaspoons maple syrup or liquid sweetener (optional, to balance the acidic lemon and spicy mustard)

- Freshly ground black pepper

- ⅓ cup fresh dill, packed and then chopped

- ½ bunch green onions (green part), sliced

- 3 stalks celery, trimmed and sliced

- ½ white onion, diced

INSTRUCTIONS

- Wash the potatoes and cut out any bad spots or eyes. Steam gently for about 10 minutes, until just fork tender through the center. Immediately run under cold water to prevent further cooking.

- For best results, refrigerate the cooked potatoes for about an hour. (This ensures they don't fall apart when slicing.)

- Quarter the potatoes and peel if desired. Place in a large bowl.

- Peel and mash the avocado in a small bowl. Add the lemon juice, mustard, paprika, Herbamare or salt, and maple syrup (if using), and stir into the avocado to create a dressing. Season with pepper to taste.

- Add the dill, green onion, celery, onion, and avocado dressing to the potatoes. Toss gently until everything is coated. Taste test and adjust seasonings if desired.

- Serve the same day, or refrigerate and serve the next day, (as the avocado darkens and breaks down quickly

3. **MINESTRONE IN MINUTES**

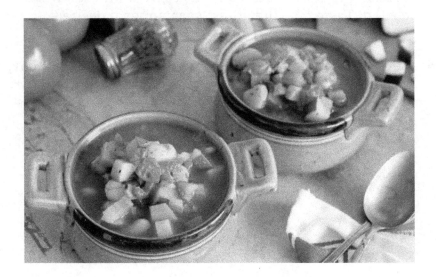

Ridiculously easy? Check. Incredibly flavorful and satisfying? Double check,This is a delicious, make-it-your-own Italian vegetable soup. Add any vegetables or beans you want to use up, or a small amount of cooked rice or pasta—just place it in the bottom of your bowl and ladle the hot soup on top. To save time, you can even use frozen mixed vegetables to replace the carrots, celery, and zucchi

INGREDIENTS

- 1 large onion, chopped
- 2 medium carrots, chopped
- 1 stalk celery, chopped
- 2 large cloves garlic, minced
- 1 (14.5-ounce) can diced tomatoes, undrained
- 1 (15.5-ounce) can cannellini beans (or other white beans), drained and rinsed

- 1 medium zucchini, diced
- 4 cups vegetable broth
- 1 teaspoon dried basil
- ½ teaspoon dried oregano
- salt and ground black pepper

INSTRUCTIONS

- Heat a large saucepan over medium heat. Place the onion, carrots, celery, and garlic into the pan and cook, stirring occasionally, until softened, about 7 minutes. Add water 1 to 2 tablespoons at a time as needed, to keep the vegetables from sticking to the pan.

- Stir in the tomatoes and their juices, beans, zucchini, and broth. Add the basil, oregano, and salt and pepper to taste. Bring to a boil, then reduce the heat to low, cover, and simmer until the vegetables are tender, about 20 minutes.

- Taste and adjust the seasonings, adding more salt and pepper if needed. Serve hot.

4. BROCOLLI SOUP

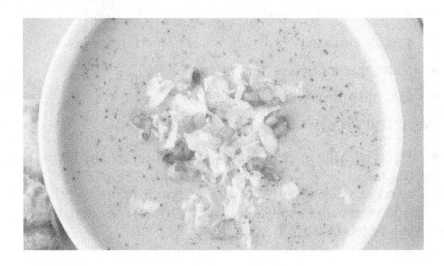

This hearty soup not only tastes great, but it's easy to make!

INGREDIENTS

- 1½ pounds Yukon gold potatoes (2 to 3 large), cut into chunks (skin on or off)
- 1 medium yellow onion, chopped
- 2 teaspoons ground coriander
- 1 teaspoon granulated garlic
- 1 teaspoon granulated onion
- 1 teaspoon no-salt poultry seasoning
- 1½ pounds broccoli (1 to 2 heads), coarsely chopped
- 3 large leaves Swiss chard, ends trimmed and coarsely chopped

INSTRUCTIONS

- Combine the potatoes, onion, coriander, granulated garlic and onion, poultry seasoning, and 6 cups water in a large soup pot, and bring to a boil.

- Reduce the heat to medium, and add the broccoli. Cook covered for about 10 minutes, until the potatoes and broccoli are tender (stirring occasionally). Stir in the chard and cook for 5 minutes more. Remove from the heat and let stand for 5 minutes.

- Blend the soup right in the pot using an immersion blender, until the soup is fairly smooth but still has some small chunks. (If you don't have an immersion blender, ladle batches of the soup into a standard blender and process gently before returning to the pot.) Serve immediately.

5. RED LENTIL DAL

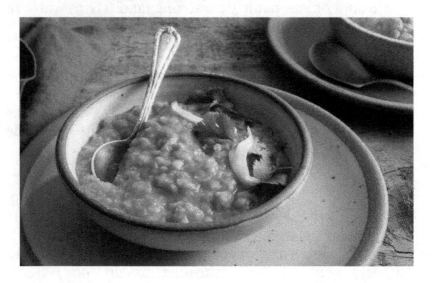

The lentils in this red lentil recipe are mushy but still intact, giving it a very traditional texture. Blend the lentils in a blender before adding the lemon juice and cilantro for a soupier texture. This is delicious served on its own, but it can also be used as the base for a variety of vegan soups Simply toss in any vegetables and some leftover cooked grains like quinoa, brown rice, millet, or pasta for a hearty one-dish meal.

INGREDIENTS

- 1½ cups red lentils, rinsed and soaked
- 1½ teaspoons peeled and grated fresh ginger
- 1 teaspoon ground coriander
- 1 teaspoon onion powder
- ½ teaspoon ground turmeric
- ½ teaspoon ground cumin
- ½ teaspoon garlic powder

- Sea salt

- 1 tablespoon fresh lemon juice (from 1 lemon)

- 1 tablespoon finely chopped fresh cilantro

- Steamed rice or whole-grain bread, for serving

INSTRUCTIONS

- Place the lentils in a saucepan and add 4 cups of water.

- Bring to a boil over high heat. Reduce the heat to medium and stir in the ginger.

- Cover the pan and simmer until the lentils are soft and have turned yellow, 15 to 20 minutes.

- Add the coriander, onion powder, turmeric, cumin, garlic powder, salt to taste, and 1 cup water if the dal is very thick. Simmer for about 10 minutes more to blend the flavors.

Stir in the lemon juice and cilantro. Taste and adjust the seasoning. Serve hot,

BAKED AND STUFFED

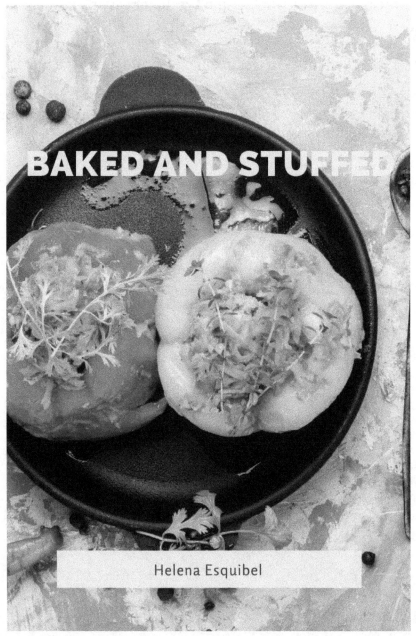

BAKED AND STUFFED

Helena Esquibel

6. <u>TWICE-BAKED SWEET POTATOES</u>

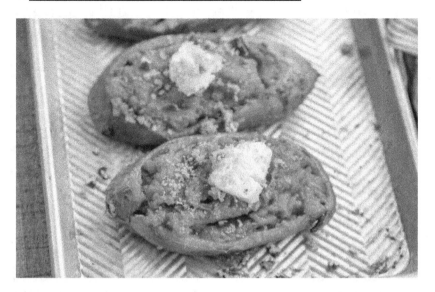

INGREDIENTS

- 4 large sweet potatoes (about 2 lbs), scrubbed
- ½ yellow onion, diced small
- ½ red bell pepper, diced small
- 2 cloves garlic, minced
- 2 teaspoons curry powder
- 1 cup frozen or fresh peas
- 1 cup cooked or canned (and drained and rinsed) chickpeas
- ½ cup toasted cashews
- ½ cup chopped fresh cilantro
- sea salt

INSTRUCTIONS

- Preheat the oven to 350°F.

- Pierce each sweet potato a few times with a fork, then place them on a baking sheet and bake until tender, 45 to 60 minutes.

- While the sweet potatoes bake, sauté the onions and bell peppers in a skillet over medium heat, stirring frequently, until the onions turn translucent and start to brown, about 8 minutes. Add the garlic and curry powder and cook for 1 more minute. Add the peas, chickpeas, cashews, and cilantro, and cook for 2 to 3 minutes to marry the flavors.

- When the sweet potatoes are tender, let them cool until they are easily handled. Cut each sweet potato in half lengthwise and scoop out all but a ½-inch wall of the flesh. Add the scooped sweet potato flesh to the skillet with the chickpea mixture. Mix well, then season with sea salt to taste.

- Spoon the filling into each of the sweet potato halves and place them back on the baking sheet. Bake until the tops of the sweet potatoes start to brown, about 25 minutes. Serve with the Sour "Cream."

7. __MILLET LOAF__

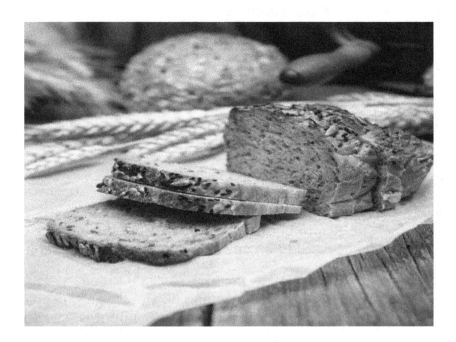

The majority of vegan "meat loaf" recipes use beans, grains, or processed soy foods and taste nothing like mom's. This hearty version includes millet, a versatile meatloaf ingredient that absorbs the flavor of whatever spices you cook with. Because millet loses its binding power as it cools, pour the mixture into the baking dish as soon as the spices are combined.

INGREDIENTS

- 2½ cups low-sodium vegetable broth or water
- ¾ cup millet
- 1 cup finely chopped onion
- 1 tablespoon snipped fresh sage
- 1 tbsp snipped fresh thyme
- 4 tablespoon garlic, minced

- ½ teaspoon freshly ground black pepper

- ⅛ teaspoon ground nutmeg

- 2 tablespoons white miso paste

- ¼ cup hot water

- ¾ cup tomato sauce or ketchup

- ¼ cup nutritional yeast (optional)

- Salt, to taste

INSTRUCTIONS

- In a medium saucepan bring broth to boiling. Stir in millet. Return to boiling; reduce heat to medium. Cover pan, and cook 20 to 25 minutes or until millet is tender.

- Meanwhile, preheat oven to 350°F. In a large saucepan cook onion over medium heat 7 to 8 minutes, stirring occasionally and adding water 1 to 2 tablespoons at a time as needed to prevent sticking. Add sage, thyme, garlic, pepper, and nutmeg; cook and stir 1 minute.

- Dissolve the miso paste in ¼ cup hot water, and stir into onion mixture. Stir in ¼ cup of the tomato sauce and nutritional yeast, if using the yeast. Stir in cooked millet. Season with salt.

- Immediately press mixture into a 9x5-inch nonstick loaf pan. Top with the remaining ½ cup tomato sauce. Bake 30 minutes or until heated through. Let stand 10 minutes before slicing.

8. <u>SMOKY LITTLE DEVILS</u>

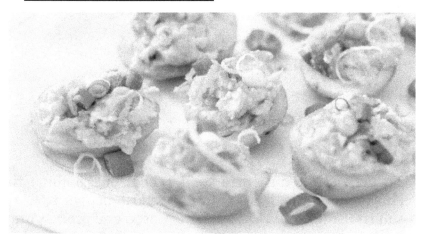

These tiny stuffed potatoes are absolutely stunning and oh so delicious as hors d'oeuvres or as the main course of a meal. Make sure the potatoes are small. Remember to keep your cool! Don't eat all of them before your guests arrive!

FOR THE HUMMUS:

- 1 (15-ounce) can no-salt-added chickpeas, drained and rinsed
- 2 large cloves 2 tablespoons fresh lemon juice
- 1½ tablespoons spicy brown mustard, or to taste
- Freshly ground black pepper, to taste
- ¼ teaspoon salt (optional; we do not use it)
- 1 cup chopped green onions (4 to 5)
- 2 teaspoons Dijon mustard, or to taste
- Zest of 1 lemon
- 1½ to 2 additional tablespoons fresh lemon juice, to taste
- ½ teaspoon ground turmeric

FOR THE DEVILS

- 12 small red potatoes (roughly the size of large walnuts or small clementines)
- Pinch of smoked paprika, for garnish
- 1 green onion, finely sliced, for garnish
- Baby kale leaves, for garnish (optional)
- Green Onion Hummus

INSTRUCTIONS

- To make Hummus, in a food processor, combine the chickpeas, garlic, lemon juice, mustard, pepper to taste, salt (if using), and 2 tablespoons water, and process until uniformly smooth.

- In a small bowl, stir together the hummus, green onions, Dijon mustard, lemon zest, additional lemon juice, and turmeric. Dollop or spread on immediately or store in an airtight container until ready to use.

- To make the Smoky Devils, set a steamer insert in a saucepan and add about 2 inches of water. Bring to a boil over high heat; then place the potatoes in the steamer basket and steam for about 20 minutes. Plunge them into cold water in a big bowl or just run cold water over them.

- Slice each potato in half. With the small end of a melon-baller or a small spoon, scoop out a hole in the center. (Save the little scooped-out potato balls to put into a salad or just pop them into your mouth!)

- Fill each hole with hummus. Sprinkle with smoked paprika. It is easiest to take a tiny bit between your fingers and sprinkle just enough for the color to show. Garnish with green onions or, for a really fun look, use a tiny baby kale leaf as a "sail" in each little potato "boat."

9. MUSHROOM-BASIL AU GRATIN

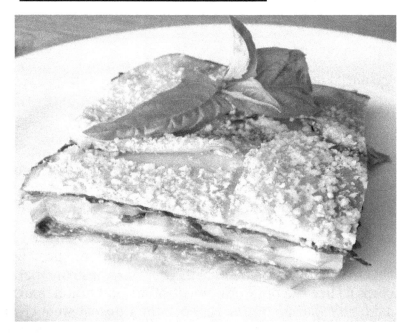

INGREDIENTS

ENTREE:

- 4-5 large Yukon potatoes, sliced thinly
- 8 large white or crimini mushrooms, sliced thinly
- 1 yellow onion, sliced thinly
- 1 bunch chard
- ½ bunch fresh basil (about 20 leaves), roughly chopped

SAUCE:

- ⅓ cup raw cashews
- 1 cup water

- ½ cup non-dairy milk

- ½ cup parsley leaves

- 2 green onions, diced

- ½ teaspoon garlic powder

INSTRUCTIONS

- In a high-speed blender, grind the cashews by themselves first; then add the water, soy milk, parsley, green onions and garlic powder and blend thoroughly. Set aside.

- To prepare the vegetables, using a mandolin slicer with the thin slicing blade (as if you were making potato chips), slice the potatoes, mushrooms and onion, and set aside in separate bowls. Remove the thickest stems from the chard leaves, and rough chop the basil; wash both and set aside.

- In a 13"x9" rectangular glass baking dish, layer vegetables in this order, starting with a thin layer of sauce in the bottom of the dish (you do not need to oil or prepare the pan): potatoes, mushrooms, onions, basil, chard, sauce. Add a second layer of vegetables and sauce, then finish with a final layer of potatoes, pouring the last bit of sauce over the top. Cover with aluminum foil and bake at 400 degrees for 35 minutes. Remove the foil and cook an additional 15 minutes until lightly browned (optional: grind some cashews on top first). Remove and let sit for at least 5 minutes before serving.

  Notes: Don't be afraid to pile the vegetables high when making your layers, as everything will condense down quite a bit while cooking. If you don't have a high-speed blender (like a Vitamix or Tribest personal blender), you may use a standard blender; just soak the cashews in the

1 cup of water for about 15 minutes first. If there are small cashew pieces in your sauce, no worries, it will still work   fine.

For a lower fat dish, leave the cashews off and decrease the water by ½ cup. The layers will not stick together as well, but the flavor will still be great. If you do not have a mandolin, just slice the vegetables by hand as thinly as you can. This dish makes great leftovers.

10. EGGPLANT ROLLATINI

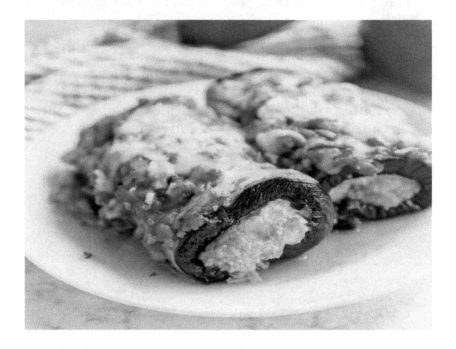

This Italian-style eggplant rollatini is typically stuffed with bread crumbs and cheeses. This version has a savory millet and spinach filling that is seasoned with fresh basil and baked before being topped with tomato sauce. This can be served on its own or with a salad or on a bed of pasta.

INGREDIENTS

- 3 whole cloves garlic, plus 5 cloves, peeled and minced
- 2 tablespoons low-sodium soy sauce
- ¼ cup low-sodium vegetable broth or <u>Vegetable Stock</u>
- 2 large eggplants, stemmed and cut lengthwise into ½ inch slices
- 1 cup millet

- Salt to taste

- 1 medium yellow onion, peeled and diced small

- 1 celery stalk, diced small

- 1 carrot, peeled and grated

- 6 cups packed chopped spinach

- ½ cup minced basil

- ¼ cup nutritional yeast, optional

- Freshly ground black pepper to taste

- 2 cups <u>Tomato Sauce</u>

INSTRUCTIONS

- Preheat the oven to 350°F.

- In a small bowl with a fork, or using a mortar and pestle, mash the 3 whole cloves of garlic with the soy sauce.

- Combine the mashed garlic mixture with the vegetable stock to make a marinade.

- Place the eggplant slices on a baking sheet and brush with some of the marinade. Bake for 10 minutes. Turn the slices over, brush with more of the marinade, and bake for another 10 to 15 minutes, until the eggplant is tender. Remove the eggplant from the oven and set aside.

- Bring 3 cups of water to a boil and add the millet and salt. Return to a boil, then reduce the heat to medium and cook, covered, for 20 minutes, or until tender.

- Place the onion, celery, and carrot in a large saucepan and sauté over medium heat for 7 to 8 minutes. Add water 1 to 2 tablespoons at a time to keep the vegetables from sticking to the pan. Add the remaining minced garlic and cook for 3 minutes. Add the spinach, basil, and nutritional yeast (if using) and season with black pepper. Cook until the spinach is wilted, then remove from the heat, add the cooked millet, and mix well.

- Spread 1 cup of the tomato sauce in the bottom of a 9 x 13-inch baking dish. Divide the millet mixture among the baked eggplant slices and roll each slice over the millet mixture. Place the eggplant rolls, seam side down, in the prepared baking dish. Cover with the remaining tomato sauce and bake, covered, for 15 minutes.

11. EGGPLANT CANNELLONI WITH BRAVO TOMATO SAUCE

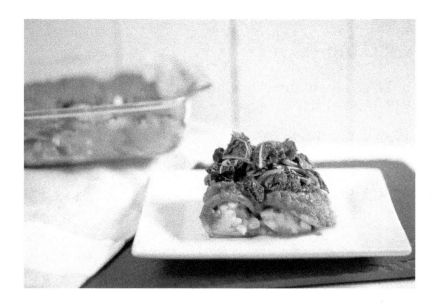

Cannelloni are pasta tubes that are round in shape. In this recipe, I use rolled eggplant instead of pasta. Choose eggplants that are large for their size. They should have shiny, firm skin that is free of soft or brown spots

INGREDIENTS

FILLING:

- 6 medium russet potatoes, peeled and cut in half widthwise
- Kernels sliced from 6 ears fresh corn, or 6 cups thawed frozen or drained canned corn
- ½ cup vegetable broth
- ½ cup unsweetened soymilk

- ½ teaspoon granulated garlic
- 1 tablespoon blanched fresh tarragon, chopped, or 1 teaspoon dried

CANNELLONI:

- 2 large eggplants, peeled and cut lengthwise into 1/8-inch-thick slices
- ½ cup vegetable broth
- ½ teaspoon granulated onion
- 4 cups Bravo Tomato Sauce

TOPPING:

- ½ cup sliced red onion
- 1 teaspoon chopped garlic
- 1 pound fresh spinach

- Cannelloni are round pasta tubes. In this recipe, I substitute rolled eggplant for the pasta. Select eggplants that are heavy for their size. They should have shiny, firm skins without any soft or brown spots.

- From Bravo! Health-Promoting Meals from The TruthNorth Kitchen

Instructions:

- Preheat the oven to 350° F.

- To make the filling, steam the potatoes until fork-tender, about 35 minutes. Transfer to a large bowl. Put half of the corn and the broth, soy milk, granulated garlic, and granulated onion in a blender and process on high speed until smooth. Spoon into the bowl with the potatoes. Add the remaining corn and the tarragon and whisk gently. (Whisking gently, rather than whipping, prevents the potatoes from getting gummy.)

- To make the cannelloni, line a rimmed baking sheet with parchment paper and arrange the eggplant on it in a single layer. Brush with the broth and sprinkle with the granulated onion. Bake for 5 minutes, then turn over and bake for 3 minutes longer. Let cool. When cool enough to handle, lay on a flat surface. Spoon one-sixth of the filling on the end of one slice and roll-up. Assemble 5 more rolls in the same fashion (to make 6 rolls in all). Put the rolls in a 13 x 9-inch baking dish, <u>pour the tomato sauce</u> over them, and bake uncovered for 15 minutes.

To make the topping, put the onion and garlic in a medium dry saucepan over medium heat and cook, stirring constantly, for 2 minutes. Add the spinach and cook, stirring occasionally, until wilted and tender, 3 to 5 minutes.

- Arrange the spinach on top of the cannelloni. Serve hot or warm.

12. SWEET POTATO, PEAR, AND BLUEBERRY FLATBREADS

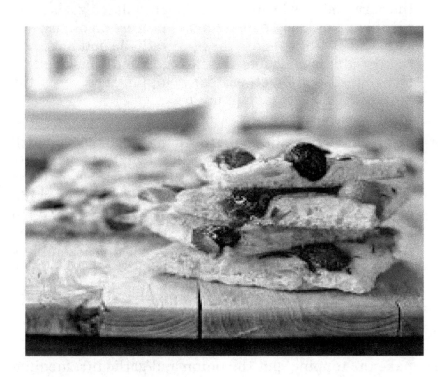

INGREDIENTS

- Cornmeal, for dusting
- 1 recipe Homemade Oil-Free Pizza Dough
- 1 cup cubed peeled sweet potato
- Sea salt and freshly ground black pepper, to taste
- 1 fresh pear, quartered and cored
- ¾ cup fresh blueberries
- 2 tablespoons chopped toasted walnuts
- 4 teaspoons pure maple syrup

- Ground cinnamon

INSTRUCTIONS

- Preheat oven to 400°F. Lightly sprinkle a large baking sheet with cornmeal.

- Divide dough into four portions. On a lightly floured surface, roll portions into 7- to 8-inch circles or 10×5-inch ovals. Transfer flatbreads to prepared pan. Bake 10 to 13 minutes or until lightly browned and set (flatbreads may puff). Let cool.

- In a small saucepan combine sweet potato and enough water to cover. Bring to boiling; reduce heat. Cover and simmer about 10 minutes or until tender. Drain and return to saucepan. Mash with a fork. Season with salt and pepper.

- Meanwhile, heat a grill pan over medium-high. Cook pear quarters about 3 minutes per cut side or until tender and light grill marks appear. Thinly slice quarters lengthwise.

- Spread sweet potato on flatbreads. Top with pear slices, blueberries, and walnuts. Drizzle with maple syrup and sprinkle with cinnamon.

13. KIWI-ORANGE FLATBREADS

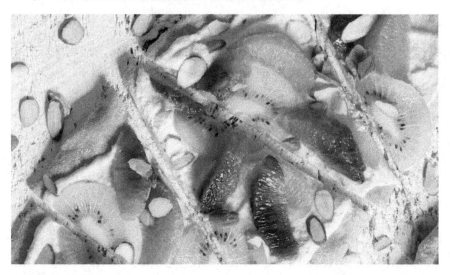

Warm homemade crusts are slathered with creamy orange cashew sauce and topped with sliced kiwis and oranges for these delectable flatbreads. If you can't find Cara Cara or blood oranges, substitute red grapefruit, navel oranges, or fresh berries.

INGREDIENTS

- Cornmeal, for dusting
- 1 recipe <u>Homemade Oil-Free Pizza Dough</u>
- ½ cup raw cashews
- ¼ cup orange juice
- ½ tsp. orange zest
- Sea salt and freshly ground black pepper, to taste
- 2 fresh blood and/or Cara Cara oranges, segmented, or 4 mandarin oranges, sectioned
- 2 fresh kiwifruits, peeled and sliced

- 2 Tbsp. toasted sliced almonds

INSTRUCTIONS

- Preheat oven to 400°F. Lightly sprinkle a large baking sheet with cornmeal.

- Divide dough into four portions. On a lightly floured surface, roll portions into 7- to 8-inch circles or 10×5-inch ovals. Transfer flatbreads to prepared pan. Bake 10 to 13 minutes or until lightly browned and set (flatbreads may puff). Let cool.

- For cashew cream, in a small bowl combine cashews and enough boiling water to cover. Let stand 1 hour. Drain. Transfer to a small food processor. Add orange juice and orange zest; cover and process until smooth and creamy. Add water, 1 tsp. at a time, and process until desired consistency. Season with salt and pepper.

- Spread cashew cream over flatbreads. Top with orange segments, kiwi slices, and almonds.

14. VEGAN BUTTERNUT SQUASH LASAGNA ROLL-UPS

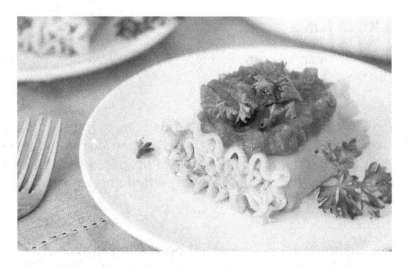

This vegan lasagna roll-up recipe is a refreshing, plant-based twist on traditionally cheesy lasagna. Butternut squash and navy beans come together to make a creamy filling that pairs well with marinara.

INGREDIENTS

- 5 cups 1-inch cubes butternut squash
- 12 whole wheat or brown rice lasagna noodles
- 3 cups cooked or canned navy beans
- 4 teaspoons sweet white miso
- 4 teaspoons well-stirred tahini
- 4 garlic cloves, minced
- 2 tablespoons nutritional yeast
- 1½ teaspoons dried basil
- 1 teaspoon dried oregano

- 1 teaspoon onion powder
- ½ teaspoon dried parsley
- Pinch red pepper flakes
- ½ teaspoon salt
- 2 tablespoons lemon juice
- 1 packed cup baby spinach, chopped
- 2½ cups marinara sauce
- Fresh parsley for garnish (optional)

INSTRUCTIONS

- Preheat the oven to 400°F. Line a large baking sheet with parchment paper and spread the squash cubes out in a single layer. Roast in the oven for 25 minutes, flip and roast for another 10 minutes, or until squash is tender and easily pierced with a fork.

- Meanwhile, bring a large pot of water to a boil. Cook the lasagna noodles according to package directions, but undercook by 1 to 2 minutes. Fill a large bowl with cold water. Drain the noodles, being careful not to tear them, and transfer them to the bowl of water to cool.

- Remove the roasted butternut squash from the oven and reduce the oven temperature to 375°F. In the bowl of a food processor, combine the squash, beans, miso, tahini, garlic, nutritional yeast, basil, oregano, onion powder, dried parsley, red pepper flakes, salt, and lemon juice; process until well combined but not completely smooth. Add the chopped spinach, and pulse until just combined.

- Spread 1½ cups of marinara sauce over the bottom of a 9x13-inch casserole dish. Drain the lasagna noodles and pat dry. Lay the noodles flat on a clean cutting board, and spread 1/3 cup of butternut filling down the center of each noodle, leaving 1 inch at each end. Keep the filling away from the sides of the noodle, as the filling will spread once rolled. Take one end of the noodle and start rolling it, gently lifting as you roll so the filling isn't pushed out. Lay the lasagne2 roll seam-side-down in the casserole dish.

- Repeat with remaining lasagna noodles and butternut filling. Keep a little space between the lasagna rolls to make it easier to remove them from the dish. Cover the lasagna rolls with the remaining marinara sauces.

- Bake, covered, at 375°F for 25 to 30 minutes. Remove from the oven and let sit for 5 minutes before serving. Serve garnished with fresh parsley

15. EASY BAKE BEAN

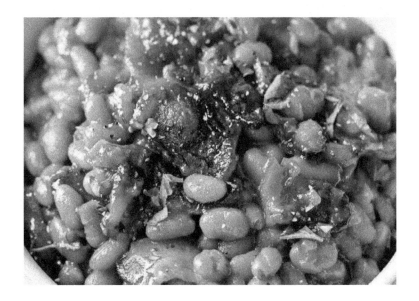

When you have homemade barbecue sauce in the fridge, you can make this dish in minutes. Because the barbecue sauce is what makes this dish, if you don't have time to make it at home, substitute a great-tasting, low-sodium sauce. Serve with roasted or grilled vegetables for a vibrant and flavorful meal.

INGREDIENTS

- 2 (15-ounce) cans pinto beans, rinsed and drained
- 2 cups Del's Basic Barbecue Sauce

INSTRUCTIONS

- Preheat the oven to 325°F.

- Combine the pinto beans and barbecue sauce in a large bowl, and mix well. Transfer the beans to an 8 × 8-inch casserole dish.

- Bake, uncovered, for 1 hour. Let stand for 5 minutes before serving.

16. GREEK STUFFED PEPPERS

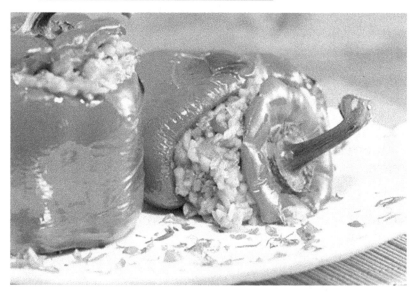

It's such a great way to use up leftover brown rice and it makes such a beautiful addition to any meal. You can also freeze these by slicing the peppers in half and storing them in air tight containers for reheating later on.

INGREDIENTS

- 6 large or 8 small bell peppers
- 1 large onion, diced
- 3 small zucchini, peeled and diced
- 3 medium carrots, peeled and diced
- 1 cup low-sodium vegetable broth
- 3 cups cooked brown rice
- 5 tablespoons tomato paste
- ¾ cup fresh parsley, chopped
- ¾ cup fresh dill, chopped
- 1 lemon, juiced

- ¼ teaspoon pepper
- ½ teaspoon Herbamare or salt

INSTRUCTIONS

- Preheat oven to 350° F.

- Cut around stem of peppers like you would cut a jack-o-lantern top, retaining the top with stem. Remove seeds carefully and wash and dry thoroughly.

- Place peppers in an oven safe dish and arrange upright and put tops back on.

- Bake at 350° F for 30 minutes.

- Meanwhile in a large non stick pan, saute onions, zucchini and carrots in vegetable broth for 5-6 minutes.

- Stir in the rice and tomato paste and coat thoroughly.

- Add parsley, dill, lemon juice, pepper and Herbamare (or salt) and stir to combine.

- When peppers are ready, take out of oven and fill with stuffing.

- Place tops back on peppers and bake for an extra 30-40 minutes until the peppers are soft.

- Serve with additional wedges of lemon and dill for garnish if desired.

17. OVEN-BAKED CHICKPEA RATATOUILLE

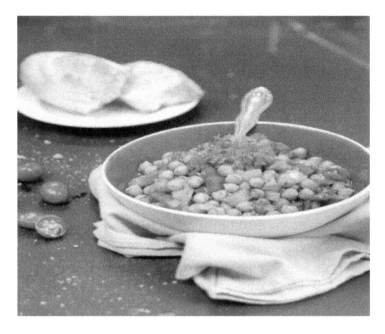

In appearance, this dish is similar to ratatouille, but it uses chickpeas and a unique spice combination. The flavors are complex, and the preparation is straightforward.

INGREDIENTS

- 3½ - 4 cups cooked chickpeas
- 1 ¼ cups red onion, finely chopped
- 3 - 4 medium-large cloves garlic, minced
- 1 28 ounce can (796-ml) diced tomatoes (see note)
- ½ cup red or orange bell pepper, diced
- 2 tablespoons apple cider vinegar
- 1 tablespoon freshly grated ginger
- 2 teaspoons pure maple syrup or agave nectar
- 2 teaspoons mustard seeds

- 2 teaspoons dried basil
- 1 teaspoon dried oregano
- ½ teaspoon dried rosemary
- 1 teaspoon sea salt
- ⅛ teaspoon allspice
- freshly ground black pepper to taste
- 2 dried bay leaves

Instructions:

- Preheat oven to 400° F.

- In a large, deep casserole dish, combine all ingredients except bay leaves. Stir through until well combined, then embed bay leaves in the mixture.

- Cover and bake for 30 minutes. Stir through, cover, and bake for another 35-45 minutes, until onions are tender and translucent (stir through once more during baking). Remove bay leaves and serve over quinoa or brown rice. Makes 4-5 servings.

Chef's Notes:

- Use regular diced tomatoes, or Italian flavored or fire-roasted for a twist.

- Try making burritos with leftovers. Spoon the mixture onto whole-grain tortillas, roll up and place in a baking dish, then bake until golden.

- This makes a large batch, but portions can be refrigerated or frozen.

VEGAN GRAIN RECIPIES

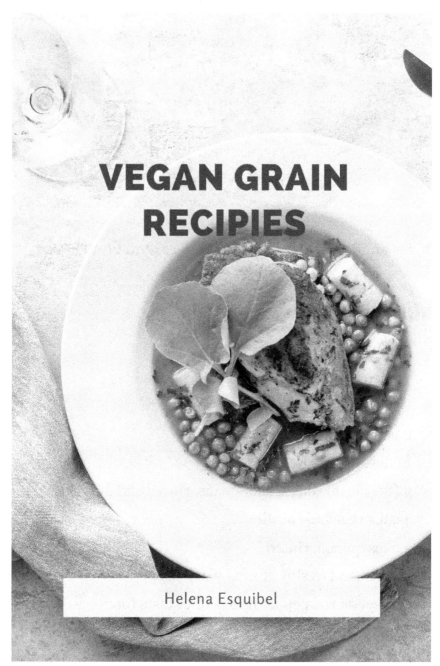

VEGAN GRAIN
RECIPIES

Helena Esquibel

18. **RED BEANS & QUINOA**

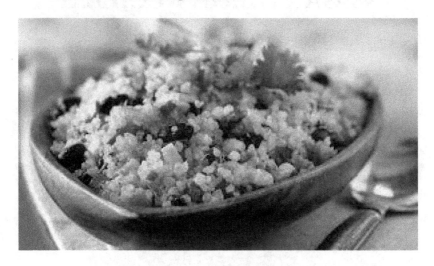

This is an ideal weeknight meal or weekend brunch dish.

INGREDIENTS

- 1 large onion, chopped
- 1 green bell pepper, seeded and chopped
- 2 stalks celery, chopped
- 2 tablespoons minced garlic
- 1 tablespoon dried thyme
- 3 (15-ounce) cans kidney beans, rinsed and drained
- 4 cups vegetable broth
- 2 cups quinoa, rinsed
- Sea salt and freshly ground black pepper
- 1 teaspoon red pepper flakes, or to taste (optional)

INSTRUCTIONS

- Place the onion, bell pepper, and celery in a large saucepan over medium-high heat. Cook, stirring occasionally and adding water 1 to 2 tablespoons at a time as needed to keep the vegetables from sticking, until the onions start to turn translucent, about 5 minutes.

- Add the garlic and thyme and cook until the garlic is softened and fragrant, about 1 minute. Add the kidney beans and vegetable broth. Bring to a boil over medium-high heat. Reduce the heat to medium-low and cook, covered, to allow the flavors to come together, about 10 minutes.

- Stir in the quinoa. Season with salt, black pepper, and red pepper flakes (if using), and simmer, covered, until the quinoa is cooked and the flavors are well blended, 12 to 15 minutes. Taste and adjust the seasoning. Serve hot

19. WILD RICE, CABBAGE AND CHICKPEA PILAF

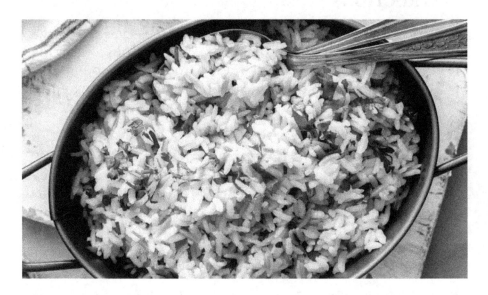

INGREDIENTS

- ½ cup wild rice
- 1 medium onion, peeled and diced small
- 1 medium carrot, peeled and grated
- 1 small red bell pepper, seeded and diced small
- 3 cloves garlic, peeled and minced
- 1 tablespoon grated ginger
- 1½ cups chopped green cabbage
- 1 cup cooked chickpeas
- 1 bunch green onions (white and green parts), thinly sliced
- 3 tablespoons chopped cilantro
- Salt and freshly ground black pepper to taste

INSTRUCTIONS

- Bring 2 cups of water to a boil in a large saucepan. Add the wild rice and bring the water back to a boil over high heat. Reduce the heat to medium and cook, covered, for 55 to 60 minutes. Drain off any excess water and set aside.

- Heat a large skillet over a medium heat. Add the onion, carrot, and red pepper and sauté the vegetables for 10 minutes. Add water 1 to 2 tablespoons at a time to keep the vegetables from sticking to the pan.

- Add the garlic and ginger and cook for another minute. Add the cabbage and cook for 10 to 12 minutes, or until the cabbage is tender. Add the chickpeas, green onions, and cilantro. Season with salt and pepper and cook for another minute to heat the chickpeas. Remove from the heat, add the cooked wild rice, and mix well.

20. <u>BURRITO BOWL</u>

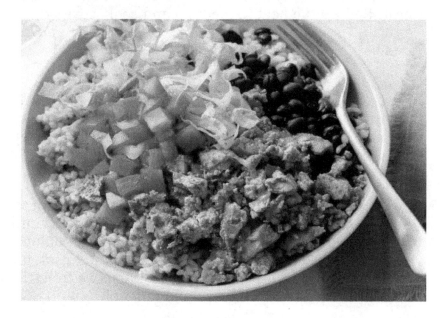

Eaten warm or cold, this simple burrito bowl is a tasty, satisfying treat!

INGREDIENTS

- Baked tortilla chips (see notes)
- 2-4 cups cooked grains (see notes)
- 2-4 cups cooked beans (see notes)
- 2-4 cups chopped romaine lettuce or steamed kale
- 2-4 chopped tomatoes
- 1-2 chopped green onions
- 1-2 cups corn kernels (see notes)
- 1 avocado, chopped
- Fresh salsas

INSTRUCTIONS

- Break a handful of the chips into pieces in the bottom of each serving bowl.

- Spoon some of the cooked grains over the chips, followed by some of the beans, then layer on the rest of the toppings: lettuce or kale, tomatoes, onions, corn, and avocado. Top with the salsa. (Use more or less of all these ingredients, as desired

21. <u>WHOLE GRAIN STUFFING WITH PECANS AND CURRANT</u>

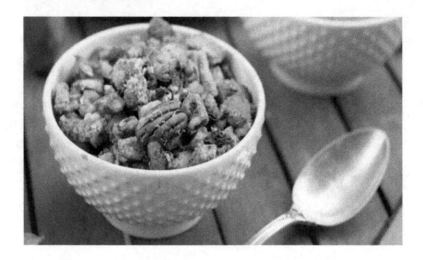

This traditional holiday recipe is enhanced with toasted pecans and currants. The earthy nuts and tart fruit add a nice twist to the otherwise mundane stuffing. Substitute half of the whole grain bread with your favorite whole grain cornbread recipe, or add fresh chopped apples for a different spin on this dish.

INGREDIENTS

- 6 cups firmly packed diced whole grain bread
- 1 medium yellow onion, diced small
- 2 stalks celery, diced small
- 1½ teaspoons fresh minced sage
- 1½ teaspoons fresh minced rosemary
- Sea salt to taste
- ½ cup toasted pecans, finely chopped
- ½ cup currants
- Freshly ground pepper to taste

- 1¼ - 1¾ cups low sodium vegetable broth

INSTRUCTIONS

- Preheat the oven to 350° F.

- Place the diced bread on a baking sheet. Bake 10 to 12 minutes, until lightly browned. Set aside.

- Sauté the onion and celery medium heat for 8 to 9 minutes. Add water 1 to 2 tablespoons at a time to keep the vegetables from sticking. Add the bread cubes and the onion mixture to a mixing bowl with the sage, rosemary, salt to taste, pecans, currants and black pepper. Mix well and drizzle the vegetable broth over the mixture to moisten.

- Transfer the mixture to a non-stick baking pan and refrigerate 1 hour for the bread crumbs to soak up all the broth.

- Bake 25 to 30 minutes, or until browned and still slightly moist.

22. CURRIED MILLET CAKES WITH CREAMY RED PEPPER CORIANDER SAUCE

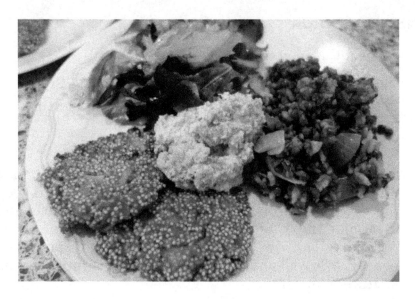

Millet, one of the oldest cultivated grains, cooks quickly and absorbs the flavor of whatever spice it is cooked with. In this dish, the versatile grain embraces Indian flavors in a dish suitable for both special occasions and weeknight dinners.

INGREDIENTS

- 3 cups Vegetable Stock, or low-sodium vegetable broth
- 1 cup millet
- 1 large yellow onion, peeled and diced small
- 4 cloves garlic, peeled and minced
- 1 tablespoon curry powder
- ½ teaspoon crushed red pepper
- 2 tablespoons mellow white miso, dissolved in ¼ cup hot water

- 2 tablespoons tomato puree
- ¼ cup nutritional yeast, optional
- Salt to taste
- 1 batch <u>Creamy Red Pepper Coriander Sauce</u>

INSTRUCTIONS

Preheat the oven to 350° F.

- Place the vegetable stock in a medium saucepan and bring to a boil over high heat. Add the millet and bring the mixture back to a boil. Reduce the heat to medium and cook, covered, for 20 minutes, or until the millet is tender.

- Place the onion in a large saucepan and sauté over medium heat for 7 to 8 minutes. Add water 1 to 2 tablespoons at a time to keep the onions from sticking to the pan. Add the garlic, curry powder, and crushed red pepper and cook for another minute. Add the miso, tomato puree, and nutritional yeast, if using, and mix well. Add the millet, season with salt, and mix well.

- Line a baking sheet with parchment paper. Using an ice cream scoop or a ¹/3-cup measure, shape the millet mixture into 12 round cakes. Place the cakes on the prepared baking sheet, and bake for 15 minutes.

- Serve

23. BASIC POLENTA

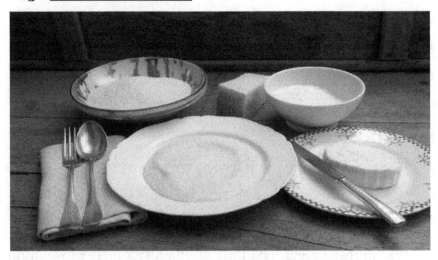

This grain dish, also known as mush or gruel, was once considered peasant food, but it has enjoyed a popular resurgence in today's culinary world. It can be served soft and creamy, or it can be allowed to set before being cut and used in a variety of dishes.

INGREDIENTS

- 1½ cups coarse cornmeal

- ¾ teaspoon salt, or to taste

INSTRUCTIONS

- Bring 5 cups of water to a boil in a large saucepan.

- Whisk in the cornmeal, a little at a time.

- Cook, stirring often, until the mixture is thick and creamy, about 30 minutes.

- Season with salt and serve, or pour the polenta into a pan and refrigerate until set, about 1 hour.

24. BARLEY AND SWEET POTATO PILAF

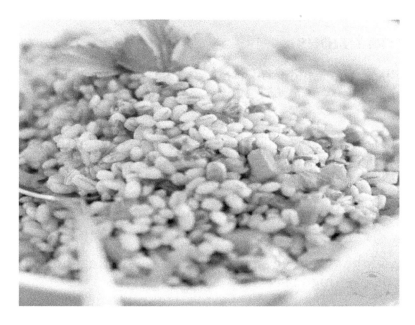

Although barley is not commonly used in pilafs, it works well as a substitute for rice. Tarragon has a milder flavor than fennel. Serve on a bed of spinach for a hearty meal.

INGREDIENTS

- 1 medium onion, peeled and chopped

- 2 cloves garlic, peeled and minced

- 3 ½ cups <u>Vegetable Stock Recipe</u> or low-sodium vegetable stock

- 1 ½ cups pearled barley

- 1 large sweet potato (about ¾ pound), peeled and diced small

- ¼ cup tarragon, minced

- Zest and juice of 1 lemon
- Salt and freshly ground black pepper to taste

INSTRUCTIONS

- Place the onion in a large saucepan and sauté over medium heat for 6 minutes.

- Add water 1 to 2 tablespoons at a time to keep the onions from sticking to the pan.

- Add the garlic and cook 3 minutes more.

- Add the vegetable stock and barley and bring the pot to a boil over high heat.

- Reduce the heat to medium and cook, covered, for 30 minutes.

- Add the sweet potato and cook for 15 minutes longer, or until the potatoes and barley are tender.

- Stir in the tarragon and lemon zest and juice, and season with salt and pepper.

SNACKS AND APPETIZERS

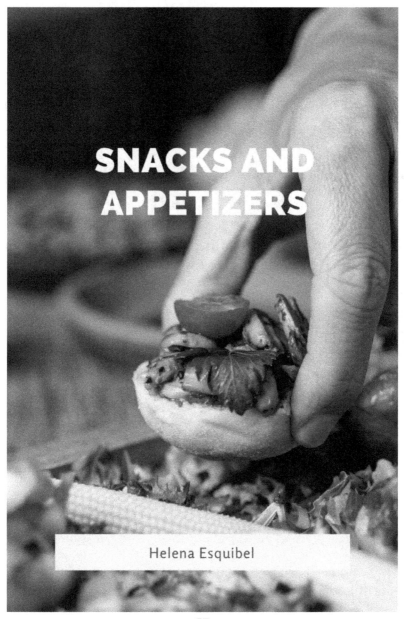

SNACKS AND
APPETIZERS

Helena Esquibel

25. __SPICY FRENCH FRIES__

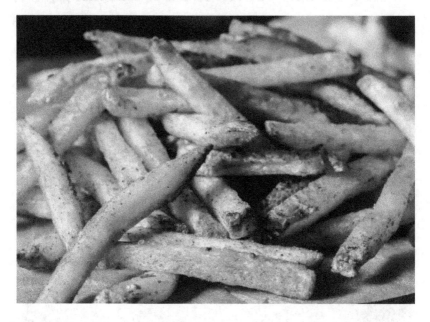

Plain baked fries are certainly tasty enough, but once in a while it's nice to spice it up, as we do here.

INGREDIENTS

- 1 tablespoon onion powder
- 1½ teaspoons garlic powder
- 1½ teaspoons sweet paprika
- 1 teaspoon ground turmeric
- 1 teaspoon ground coriander
- ¼ teaspoon cayenne pepper
- Sea salt
- 1½ pounds russet potatoes (3 or 4 medium-small), scrubbed and cut into 1-inch-thick wedges

- 2 tablespoons fresh lemon juice (from 1 lemon)
- Ketchup and Dijon mustard, for serving (optional)

INSTRUCTIONS

- Preheat the oven to 450°F. Line a baking sheet with parchment paper.

- Place a steamer basket in a large pot and add about 2 inches of water. Place the potatoes in the steamer, cover and steam on high heat for 10 minutes. The potatoes will be about 75 percent cooked.

- In the meantime, in a medium bowl, stir together the onion powder, garlic powder, paprika, turmeric, coriander, cayenne, lemon juice and salt to taste.

- Transfer the potatoes to the bowl with spices and toss gently but well to coat the potatoes evenly. Arrange the potato wedges on the baking sheet, leaving plenty of room between them.

- Bake for 20 to 25 minutes.

- Serve the fries hot, with ketchup and Dijon mustard for dipping, if desired.

26. <u>CHEESY" VEGGIE PIZZETTES</u>

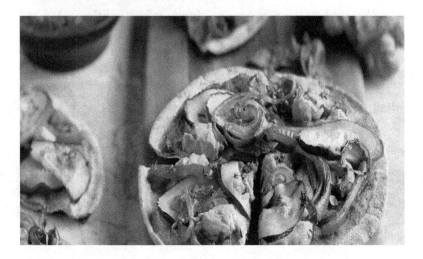

These mini pizzas are ideal for parties. Pita bread works well as a pizza crust because it cooks quickly and comes in the perfect size for individual pizzas or appetizer-size slices. The cheesy bean spread serves as a good substitute for nut-based cheese and adds a nice savory flavor to the dish. Because pita bread does not bake for as long as a traditional crust, sauté the vegetables ahead of time so they are perfectly cooked when they come out of the oven. You can also sauté the vegetables and spread the day before to make assembly easier.

INGREDIENTS

PIZZETTES

- 1 red onion, thinly sliced (2 cups)
- 1 zucchini, cut into long diagonal slices (1 cup)
- 1 red bell pepper, cut into thin strips (1 cup)
- 6 whole-wheat pita breads

- 1 ½ cups store-bought pizza or marinara sauce
- 2 tablespoons fresh basil, finely chopped

CHEESY BEAN SPREAD

- 1 (15-ounce) can white beans, drained and rinsed
- ¼ cup nutritional yeast
- 1 clove garlic, minced (½ teaspoon)
- 2 teaspoons white wine vinegar
- 1 dash crushed red pepper flakes
- Sea salt
- Freshly ground black pepper

INSTRUCTIONS

- Preheat the oven to 400°F. Line a baking sheet with parchment paper.

- Combine the onions, zucchini, and bell peppers in a skillet and sauté over medium heat, stirring frequently, for about 10 minutes or until the onions start to turn golden brown. Add water 1 to 2 tablespoons at a time as needed, to keep the vegetables from sticking to the pan.

- Place the pitas on the prepared baking sheet and bake for 5 minutes.

- Combine the beans, nutritional yeast, garlic, vinegar, and ¼ cup water in a food processor. Puree until smooth. Add pepper flakes; mix well, then season with salt and pepper to taste. Set aside.

- Remove the baking sheet from the oven and flip the pitas over.

- Spread 2 tablespoons of marinara sauce over each pita. Dot the pitas with spoonfuls of the bean spread.

- Layer the vegetables on top. Sprinkle with some basil and bake for 20 minutes.

- Remove from the heat. Slice into quarters and serve warm.

27. CRISPY BUFFALO CAULIFLOWER BITES

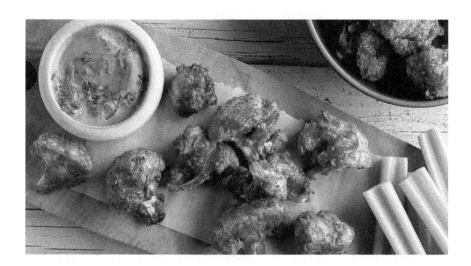

You will not need to add salt as the sauces have enough salt to season them. Either a smoky barbecue sauce or Frank's hot sauce would work well, but if you are like me and prefer sweet and spicy, then try a little bit of both. Serve with ranch or Caesar dressing on the side if you wish, or whip up a batch of Spinach Ranch Dip. Note: The buffalo cauliflower bites will get softer once they are coated with the sauce, so hold off tossing until the very last minute

INGREDIENTS

- ⅔ cup brown rice flour
- 2 tablespoons almond flour
- 1 tablespoon tomato paste
- 2 teaspoons garlic powder
- 2 teaspoons onion powder
- 2 teaspoons smoked paprika
- 1 teaspoon dried parsley

- 1 head cauliflower, cut into 2-inch florets
- ⅓ cup Frank's hot sauce or barbecue sauce
- <u>Spinach Ranch Dip</u>

INSTRUCTIONS

- Preheat oven to 450°F. Line 2 baking sheets with parchment paper.

- Combine the brown rice flour, almond flour, tomato paste, garlic powder, onion powder, paprika, parsley, and ⅔ cup of water in a blender. Puree until the batter is smooth and thick. Transfer to a bowl and add the cauliflower florets; toss until the florets are well coated with the batter.

- Arrange the cauliflower in a single layer on the prepared baking sheets, making sure that the florets do not touch one another. Bake for 20 to 25 minutes, until crisp on the edges. They will not get crispy all over while still in the oven.

- Remove from the heat and let stand for 3 minutes to crisp up a bit more. Transfer to a bowl and drizzle with the sauce. Serve immediately.

28. BANANA BLUEBERRY BARS

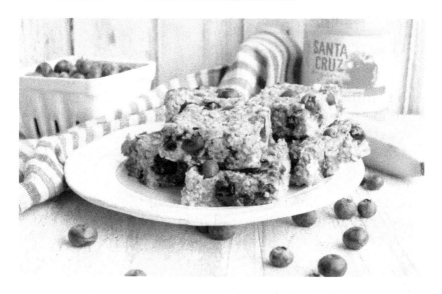

This delectable bar is ideal for breakfast, a snack, or dessert. It's high in starch, which provides long-lasting energy, and unrefined sugars, which provide a healthy sweetness. You can enjoy a tasty treat while also benefiting your body!

INGREDIENTS

- 1 cup dates, pitted and halved
- 1½ cups apple juice
- 3 cups rolled oats, divided
- ¾ teaspoon ground cinnamon
- ¼ teaspoon ground nutmeg
- 1 ½ tablespoons baking powder
- 1 large or 2 small ripe bananas
- 1 teaspoon vanilla extract

- 1 cup fresh blueberries (frozen also works)
- ½ cup walnuts

INSTRUCTIONS

- In a small bowl, soak the dates in the apple juice for 10 to 15 minutes. Preheat the oven to 375°F. Line a 9x9-inch baking pan with parchment paper, making sure the sides are covered. Cut slits in the corners of the paper so that it overlaps and lies flat.

- In a medium bowl, combine 2 cups of the rolled oats with the cinnamon, nutmeg, and baking powder. Mix and set aside.

- Place the remaining 1 cup of rolled oats, the bananas, and the vanilla extract into a blender. Remove the dates from the apple juice and set aside. Strain the juice, add it to the blender, and blend until creamy.

- Add the dates to the blender, and pulse a few times until the dates are in small pieces.

- Pour the banana mixture into the dry ingredient bowl. Mix well. Stir in the blueberries and walnuts.

- Using a spatula, pour the batter into the baking pan. Bake for 30 to 35 minutes, or until a toothpick inserted into the center comes out clean.

- Cool at room temperature for 5 to 10 minutes before cutting and serving.

29. YAMADILLAS

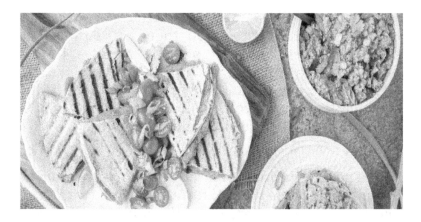

This tasty bar is ideal for breakfast, a snack, or dessert. It contains starch, which provides long-lasting energy, as well as unrefined sugars, which provide a healthy sweetness. You can enjoy a tasty treat while also supporting your body!

INGREDIENTS

- 2 pounds garnet yams, peeled and diced
- 2 tablespoons vegetable broth
- 2 tablespoons chopped green chiles
- 2 teaspoons fresh lime juice
- 1 teaspoon minced chipotle peppers in adobo sauce
- ¾ teaspoon ground cumin
- ½ teaspoon minced garlic
- 1 can (15 ounces) black beans, drained and rinsed
- 8 whole-wheat tortillas
- Fresh salsa of your choice
- Pea Guacamole

INSTRUCTIONS

- Put the yams in a stainless-steel saucepot with enough water to cover. Bring to a boil, then reduce the heat and simmer, covered, until soft, about 12 minutes. Drain the water and add the vegetable broth to the yams. Mash with a potato masher until quite smooth, then stir in the green chiles, lime juice chipotle, cumin, and garlic. Mix well, stir in the black beans, and mix again.

- Heat a nonstick griddle or large skillet over medium heat. Spread some of the yam mixture on half of a tortilla, then fold it over and flatten. Place the folded tortilla on the griddle and cook it for about 2½ minutes on each side, flipping several times to make sure it doesn't burn. Repeat with the yam mixture and tortillas. Serve topped with salsa and/or guacamole.

Note: This kid-friendly recipe makes quite a large amount. However, Yamadillas store well overnight in the refrigerator

30. MEXICAN 10-LAYER DIP

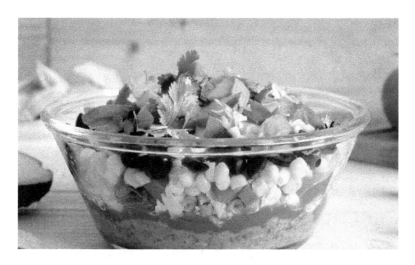

INGREDIENTS

- 4 corn tortillas
- ½ (14-ounce) package extra-firm silken tofu, drained
- 2 tablespoons fresh lemon juice
- 1 tablespoon red wine vinegar
- 1 pinch cayenne pepper (optional)
- sea salt
- 1 (15-ounce) can refried black beans (1½ cups)
- ¼ teaspoon garlic powder
- ¼ teaspoon ground cumin
- ¼ teaspoon dried oregano
- 1 cup salsa
- 1 cup shredded lettuce

- 2 scallions (white and green parts), thinly sliced
- 1 tomato, cut into small dice
- ½ cup fresh or frozen (and thawed) corn
- ½ avocado, diced (optional)
- 1 tablespoon seeded and sliced jalapeño (optional)
- 1 tablespoon finely chopped fresh cilantro (optional)
- ¼ cup sliced black olives

INSTRUCTIONS

- Preheat the oven to 350°F. Cut the tortillas into bite-size triangles and bake them on a baking sheet until crisp, 20 minutes.

- Meanwhile, combine the drained tofu, lemon juice, red wine vinegar, and cayenne pepper (if using) in a blender; season with salt to taste. Purée until smooth. Chill the tofu "sour cream" until ready to use.

- Combine the refried beans, garlic powder, cumin, and oregano in a saucepan and cook until heated through, about 5 minutes. Add 1 to 2 tablespoons of water if needed to help combine.

- Spread the beans in the base of a serving dish. Top with the salsa, followed by the lettuce, scallions, tomatoes, corn, and tofu sour cream, along with any optional ingredients. Scatter sliced olives over the dip, then serve with tortilla chips.

Pasta & Noodles

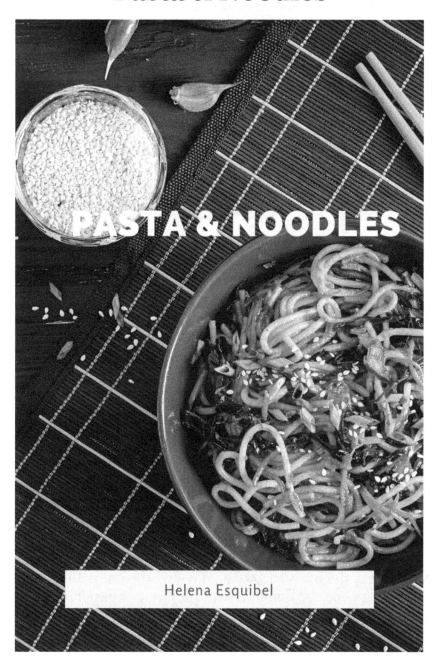

PASTA & NOODLES

Helena Esquibel

31. SPAGHETTI WITH ROASTED TOMATOES, CHICKPEAS, AND BASIL

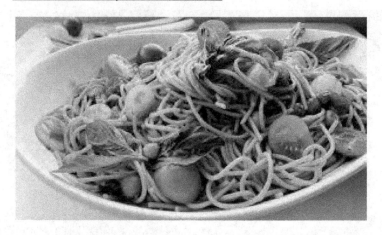

Roasting vegetables is a simple way to add flavor to a dish, and yes, you can do it without using any oil—the results are delicious

INGREDIENTS

- 1 pound cherry tomatoes
- 2 teaspoons granulated garlic
- Sea salt and freshly ground black pepper
- 12 ounces whole-grain spaghetti
- 1 (15-ounce) can chickpeas, rinsed and drained
- 1 cup chopped fresh basil

INSTRUCTIONS

- Preheat the oven to 350°F. Have ready a nonstick baking sheet or line one with parchment paper.

- Bring a large pot of water to a boil.

- Cut the tomatoes in half and place them in a bowl. Sprinkle them with the granulated garlic and salt and pepper to taste. Spread them on the baking sheet in a single layer. Roast the tomatoes until they start to shrivel, 30 to 35 minutes. Remove from the oven and set aside.

- During the last 10 minutes that the tomatoes are roasting, add the pasta to the boiling water and cook according to the package instructions. Drain the pasta, reserving about 1 cup of the pasta cooking water. Transfer the pasta to a bowl. Add the chickpeas, the roasted tomatoes, the basil, and as much of the reserved cooking water as desired to moisten, and mix well. Season to taste with salt and pepper. Serve hot.

32. <u>WHITE BEANS WITH GREENS, GARLIC AND TOMATO</u>

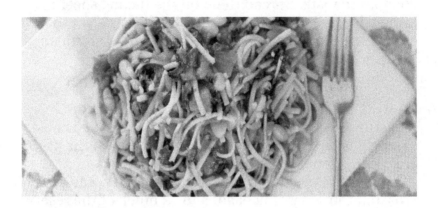

INGREDIENTS

- 1 cup white beans, soaked (see notes)*
- 1 medium onion, diced
- 6 cloves garlic, minced, half reserved
- ½ to ⅔ cup low-sodium vegetable broth
- 1 bunch greens such as kale or collards, chopped, to equal 4-6 cups
- 3 cups diced heirloom tomatoes or 1 large can unsalted diced tomatoes, drained
- Pinch of red pepper flakes, or diced hot pepper, if desired
- ½ teaspoon salt (optional)
- Black pepper, to taste

INSTRUCTIONS

Pressure Cooker Method:

Drain the beans and set aside. Heat the pressure cooker

over medium heat. Add the onion and sauté for 2 to 3 minutes. Add the garlic and sauté another minute. Add the beans and broth and lock the lid on the cooker. Bring to high pressure over high heat and then reduce the heat. Cook for 5 minutes. Remove from the heat and let the pressure come down naturally. Carefully open the lid, tilting it away from you.

Add the greens and stir. Lay the tomatoes on top of the green and beans mixture. Add the pepper flakes or hot pepper now, if using, along with the remaining garlic. Bring to high pressure again for 2 minutes. Remove from the heat and let the pressure come down naturally. Carefully open the lid and add salt and pepper, to taste. Serve hot over quinoa, other whole grain or pasta or as a side dish.

- **Stovetop Method:**

  Dry sauté the onions and half the garlic and then add the beans and broth to cover (it will be closer to 1 cup or more). Cook, simmering, until the beans are done, adding liquid as necessary to keep beans covered. Drain off most of the broth, leaving about ¼ cup in the pot.

  Add the greens, tomatoes, pepper flakes, if using, and the remaining garlic. Simmer for up to 10 minutes until the greens are cooked and the tomatoes start to break down. Season to taste. Serve hot over quinoa, other whole grain or pasta or as a side dish.

  Notes: If fresh shelling beans are available, use them. If not, soak your beans overnight or do a quick soak and then cook them quickly in the pressure cooker. No, pressure cooker? It takes much longer on the stovetop but can be done.

33. RIP'S PASTA PRIMAVERA

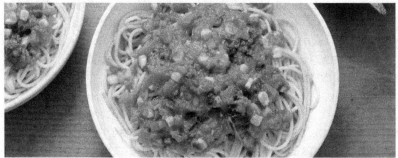

This pasta dish contains no bouillon or other meat. It's colorful, hearty, and delicious, and it's a great way to get some greens into your evening meal. It also makes excellent leftovers.

INGREDIENTS

- 1 red onion, chopped
- 1 clove garlic, minced
- 1 can corn, rinsed and drained
- 1 jalapeno pepper, minced (remove seeds to reduce heat)
- 1 green or red bell pepper, seeded and chopped
- 1 bunch fresh kale, rinsed and chopped
- 1 can diced tomatoes
- 1 large jar pasta sauce
- 16 ounces whole-grain spaghetti, cooked
- ½ cup raw cashews, finely ground

INSTRUCTIONS

- Sauté the onion, garlic, and corn in a large skillet on medium heat for 5 minutes. Add the jalapeno, bell pepper, and kale to the skillet and cook for 3 minutes. Add the diced tomatoes and pasta sauce to the vegetables. Ladle the sauce over the pasta and top with the cashews.

34. ROASTED TOMATO AND CANNELLINI BEAN PASTA

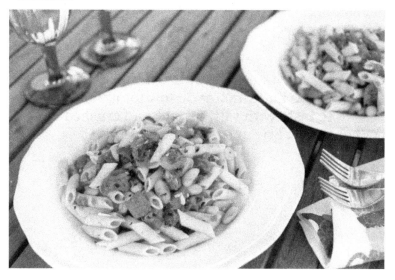

This recipe is so easy to put together and can easily be doubled

INGREDIENTS

- ½ pound whole wheat or brown rice penne pasta
- 2 tablespoons low-sodium vegetable stock or water
- 6 – 8 cloves garlic, chopped
- 1 13.4-ounce box cannellini beans, rinsed and drained
- 1 15.5-ounce can fire roasted tomatoes
- salt and pepper to taste
- crushed red pepper flakes to taste

INSTRUCTIONS

- In a large pot, cook pasta in boiling water until al dente. Set aside.

- In a medium pot, sauté garlic in vegetable stock or water over medium heat for 2-3 minutes. Stir in beans and tomatoes and simmer on low for about 20 minutes. Season to taste with salt, pepper and crushed red pepper flakes. Stir in pasta and serve.

35. MEDITERRANEAN VEGETABLE SPAGHETTI

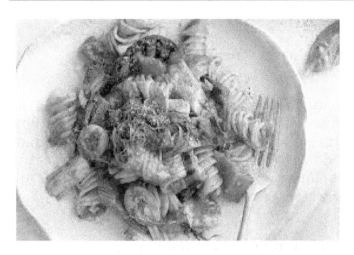

INGREDIENTS

- 10 ounces brown rice spaghetti
- 1 red bell pepper, cubed small
- 1 yellow bell pepper, cubed small
- 2 plum tomatoes, sliced into eighths (discard the seeds)
- Salt
- ½ jalapeño (optional)
- 2 tablespoons dried herbes de Provence
- 2 tablespoons tomato purée
- 2 tablespoons apple cider vinegar or juice of 1 lime
- 12 cherry tomatoes, quartered
- 1 zucchini, halved then sliced into thin half-rounds
- 1 bunch spinach, chopped
- Handful of black olives

INSTRUCTIONS

- Bring the pasta water to a boil.

- Place the chopped peppers, plum tomatoes, salt, jalapeño (optional) and herbes de Provence into a saucepan. Add ¼ cup water and allow the mix to simmer and gently cook down to form the sauce. If the liquid dries up before the tomatoes and peppers start to release their juice, add more water, 1 tablespoon at a time.

- After a few minutes, add the tomato purée and the apple cider vinegar or lime juice.

- Cook the spaghetti according to package directions.

- Once the tomato and peppers begin to meld into a sauce, add the cherry tomatoes, zucchini slices, and spinach. Mix well and cook for about 5 to 7 minutes.

- Drain the pasta, then stir the pasta, olives, and an extra sprinkling of herbes de Provence into the sauce

36. FETTUCCINE WITH GRILLED ASPARAGUS, PEAS, AND LEMON

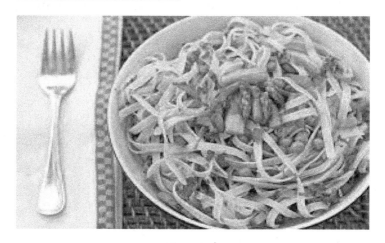

With the lightness of lemons and parsley, asparagus and peas combine to make a beautiful dish that is suitable for both lunch and dinner.

INGREDIENTS

- 6-8 stalks asparagus
- 2 cloves garlic, minced
- Juice of 1 lemon, about 2 tablespoons
- Pinch of coarse sea salt
- Water
- 6 ounces fettuccine
- 2 tablespoons minced parsley
- 1 cup peas

INSTRUCTIONS

- Toss the asparagus in the garlic, lemon juice, and salt.

- Grill the asparagus until it just starts to develop a few blackened spots. The asparagus should still have some crispness to it.

- Cut the asparagus into 2-inch pieces.

- Bring the water to a boil.

- Boil the pasta until it is al dente.

- Toss the cooked pasta with the asparagus, parsley, and peas.

37. **PONZU NOODLE SALAD**

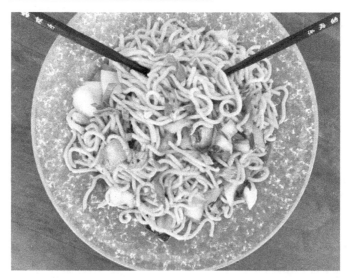

Ponzu is a popular Japanese soy and citrus sauce. Dress up simple vegetable and rice dishes with it, or use it as a sauce for stir-fries. When snow peas and cilantro are in season in the spring, make this dish. Brown rice noodles are widely available in supermarkets, natural food stores, and online.

INGREDIENTS

- 1 pound brown rice noodles

- ½ pound snow peas, trimmed and cut into matchsticks

- 3 medium carrots, peeled and cut into matchsticks

- 3 green onions (white and green parts), cut into ¾-inch pieces

- ½ cup coarsely chopped cilantro

- ½ cup Ponzu Sauce

- ½ teaspoon crushed red pepper flakes, optional

INSTRUCTIONS

- Cook the brown rice noodles according to package directions, adding the snow peas and carrots during the last minute of cooking.

- Drain and rinse the mixture until cooled, and place it in a large bowl.

- Add the green onions, cilantro, ponzu sauce, and crushed red pepper flakes, if using.

- Mix well before serving.

38. VELVETY MACARONI

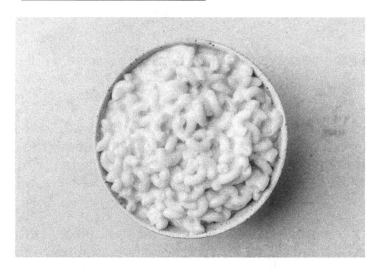

INGREDIENTS

- 1 butternut squash
- 2 medium broccoli heads
- 2½ cups dry brown rice pasta
- 4 garlic cloves
- ½ cup almond, coconut or flax seed milk
- 3 tablespoons nutritional yeast
- sea salt
- 1 tablespoon garlic powder
- parsley flakes
- pepper

INSTRUCTIONS

- Bake the butternut squash whole and unpeeled in the oven on 350°F for exactly 30 minutes. Over-baking may cause problems with the preparation later.

- Separate the broccoli into small florets and cut the broccoli stems into small pieces.

- Boil the pasta as instructed on the package while being careful not to overcook it.

- The squash should be ready by now and will peel easily after baking. Cut the squash in half and remove the seeds. Cut the squash into smaller pieces and steam it covered with the 4 garlic cloves for 10 minutes.

- In a separate pot add the broccoli stem pieces with a bit of water and steam it covered for five minutes. After five minutes, add the broccoli florets and continue steaming covered for 3-4 minutes. Drain the water from the broccoli.

- Drain the water from the butternut squash and remove it from the flame. Add the plant-based milk of choice, nutritional yeast, sea salt and garlic powder* to the pot and blend it well with an immersion blender (or in a regular blender) until it is smooth and creamy. Once smooth, add the parsley flakes and pepper to the creamy butternut and mix it with a spoon.

- Bring the creamy sauce to a very gentle low boil and add the pasta and broccoli while mixing very gently with a wooden spoon.

    Notes: You may want to use less garlic powder than what is listed since I prefer this dish pungent with garlic.

39. **PASTA PRIMAVERA**

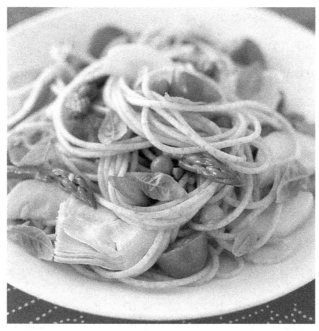

Pasta primavera is related to, and most likely derived from, traditional Italian dishes. However, this is a North American dish that originated in Nova Scotia and was brought to New York City in the early 1970s. This dish is typically high in fat and cholesterol when made with olive oil or alfredo. Fortunately, this version keeps the fat to a minimum and is completely healthy!

INGREDIENTS

- 12 ounces quinoa penne
- 3 cups broccoli, chopped
- 2 cups carrots, diced
- 1 onion, diced
- 1 cup red bell pepper, diced
- 1½ tablespoon garlic granules

- 2 cups low-sodium vegetable broth
- ½ cup raw cashews
- 1 cup soy milk
- ½ cup oat flour
- 2 cups green peas
- ¼ teaspoon black pepper
- 2 teaspoons dried basil or 2 tablespoons fresh
- 2 teaspoons dried oregano or 2 tablespoons fresh
- 1 cup cherry tomatoes, halved

INSTRUCTIONS

- In a medium pot, bring water to a boil. Then add the pasta and cook according to the directions on the box. When the pasta is slightly al dente, remove from heat, drain, and set aside. While pasta cooks, in a large sauté pan, sweat (see chef's note below) the broccoli, carrots, onion, red pepper, and garlic on medium heat for 10 minutes. Keep them covered and stir occasionally. Then stir in the vegetable broth and simmer for another 10 minutes.

- Grind the cashews in a spice grinder to form a cashew powder. A coffee grinder or blender would also work. Either way, make sure the appliance is completely dry.

- Stir in the soy milk, oat flour and cashew powder. Make sure to stir occasionally to prevent the oats from clumping together. Add the peas, black pepper, and dried herbs. Simmer for 10 minutes, continuing to stir occasionally, until the oats and cashews create a creamy sauce. Mix in the pasta and tomatoes. Best served right away. Also delicious chilled as a pasta salad.

Notes:

Sweating is a mix of sautéing and steaming. The idea is the water will come out or "sweat" from the veggies, which creates enough moisture so that no added liquid is needed. To sweat an item, put the cut veggie in a sauté pan without oil or water over medium heat. Keep the pan covered and stir frequently. Do this until the item is cooked to desired frequency. If the pan is becoming dry or veggie starts to stick to the bottom of pan, add a little bit of water or vegetable broth. You can also turn down the heat.

Because you are grinding the cashews and using oat flour, they will be slightly coarse and you will likely see specks of these two within the cream sauce. If this bothers you, you could try substituting a more refined thickening agent, such as store-bought rice flour or potato starch.

If you are using fresh herbs, add them in the last step when you are mixing in the pasta and tomatoes.

40. <u>THAI GREEN CURRY RICE</u>

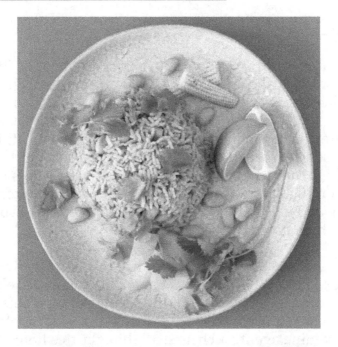

This dish calls for mild Thai green curry paste, which can be found in Asian markets, natural food stores, and some supermarkets. For a spicier version, replace the green curry paste with red curry paste, or serve with hot sauce on the side. Use Thai purple rice instead of brown rice for a more colorful dish."

- 2 cups cooked cannellini beans, or 1 (15-ounce) can, drained and rinsed

INSTRUCTIONS

- Place the cooked spaghetti in a large bowl and add the pesto. Stir well, adding enough of the reserved cooking liquid to achieve a creamy sauce. Add the beans and toss well.

- the chopped green onion and chopped peanuts.

DESSERTS

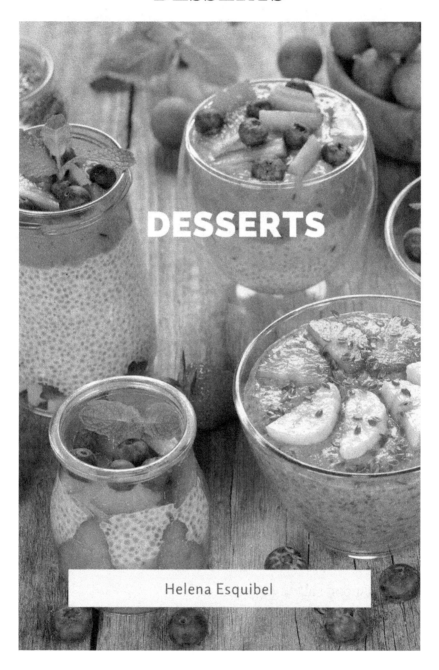

DESSERTS

Helena Esquibel

41. **CRANBERRY-ORANGE BISCOTTI**

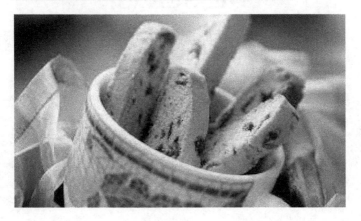

INGREDIENTS

1. ⅓ cup fresh orange juice

2. 2 tablespoons ground flaxseeds

3. ¾ cup dry sweetener (use evaporated cane juice or cane sugar)

4. ¼ cup unsweetened applesauce

5. ¼ cup almond butter

6. 1 teaspoon pure vanilla extract

7. 1⅔ cups whole-wheat pastry flour

8. 2 tablespoons cornstarch

9. 2 teaspoons baking powder

10. ½ teaspoon ground allspice

11. ½ teaspoon salt

12. ¾ cup fruit-sweetened dried cranberries

INSTRUCTIONS

13. Line a baking sheet with parchment paper or a Silpat baking mat. Preheat the oven to 350° F.

14. In a large mixing bowl, use a fork to vigorously mix together orange juice and flaxseeds until frothy. Mix in the dry sweetener, applesauce, almond butter, and vanilla.

15. Sift in the flour, cornstarch, baking powder and allspice, then add the salt and mix until well combined. Knead in the cranberries using your hands because the dough will be stiff.

16. On the prepared baking sheet, form the dough into a rectangle about 12 inches long by 3 to 4 inches wide. Bake for 26 to 28 minutes, or until lightly puffed and browned. Remove the sheet from the oven and let cool for 30 minutes.

17. Turn the oven temperature up to 375° F. With a heavy, very sharp knife, slice the biscotti into ½-inch-thick slices. The best way to do this is in one motion, pushing down; don't "saw" the slices or they may crumble. Lay the slices down on the cookie sheet and bake for 10 to 12 minutes, flipping the slices halfway through. Allow to cool for a few minutes on the baking sheet before transferring the slices to cooling racks.

42. CHOCOLATE CHIP PUMPKIN MUFFINS

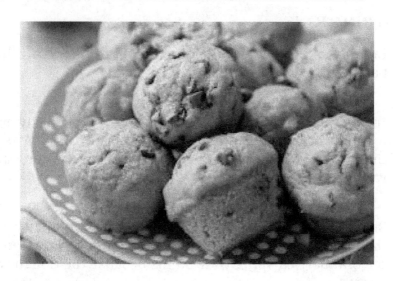

INGREDIENTS

18. 1 medium banana, mashed

19. 1 (15-ounce) can pumpkin puree

20. ¼ cup pure maple syrup

21. 1 teaspoon vanilla extract

22. 2 cups whole oat flour

23. ½ teaspoon baking soda

24. ½ teaspoon baking powder

25. ½ teaspoon salt

26. 1 teaspoon ground cinnamon

27. ½ teaspoon ground nutmeg

28. ¼ teaspoon ground ginger

29. 1 cup grain-sweetened dairy-free chocolate chips

INSTRUCTIONS

30. Preheat oven to 375°F. In a large bowl, combine mashed banana, pumpkin puree, maple syrup, and vanilla.

31. In a small bowl, combine oat flour, baking soda, baking powder, salt, cinnamon, nutmeg, and ginger. Transfer mixture to large bowl and mix together gently until well combined. Avoid over-mixing to prevent toughness in the final product. Fold in chocolate chips.

32. Spoon batter into silicon muffin cups and bake for 20 minutes or until the muffins are lightly browned. Remove muffins from the oven and let cool for 5 minutes. Store muffins in an airtight container

43. <u>BLACKBERRY-PEACH COBBLER</u>

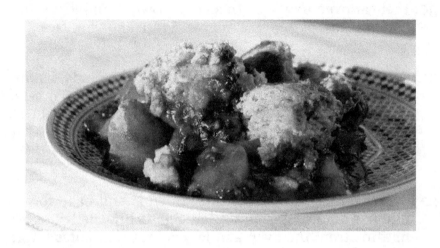

INGREDIENTS

FRUIT

33. 1- 1 ½ cups pitted and sliced fresh or frozen peaches (about 3 large peaches)

34. 2 cups blackberries

FRUIT SAUCE

35. 3 medjool dates, pitted, chopped, and soaked in water (to cover) for about 30 minutes

36. 2 tablespoon lime or lemon juice

37. ½ cup water (can use date soak water)

38. ½ teaspoon allspice

39. ¼ cup oat flour

TOPPING

40. 1-1 ½ cups rolled oats, ground into flour (or oat or other type of pre-ground flour)

41. ½ large, ripe banana, sliced

42. 3 dates, pitted, chopped, and soaked in water (to cover) for about 30 minutes

43. ½ cup plant-based milk

44. ¼ teaspoon ground allspice

45. 1-1 ½ teaspoons baking powder

46. 1 teaspoon vanilla extract

INSTRUCTIONS

47. Preheat oven to 375° F. Put the 6 dates (3 for the Fruit Sauce and 3 for the Topping) into 2 separate dishes to soak.

48. For the filling: Place peaches and blackberries into a large bowl. Set aside.

49. For the fruit sauce: Blend the dates, lime or lemon juice, water, allspice and flour in a blender until smooth. Pour into the bowl of fruit and toss. Pour the fruit mixture into a baking dish and spread out evenly. You can use most sizes of baking dishes; I use a large ceramic pie pan, but a 9x9" or a 9x13" square pan would also work, just keep in mind that the fruit and the topping will be spread out more thinly with a larger pan. (No treatment is necessary for the pan.)

50. For the topping: Using your blender again, blend the banana, dates, and non-dairy milk together until smooth.

Transfer this mixture to a bowl and add the oat flour, allspice, baking powder and vanilla extract. Mix with a fork until the texture is somewhere between dough and batter (fairly thick). Spread the topping over the fruit filling evenly, or drop by spoonfuls, leaving gaps of fruit between. Cook at 375 degrees for between 25 and 30 minutes, or until topping is lightly browned. Let sit for at least 10 minutes before serving.

44. <u>NO-BAKE CRANBERRY PEAR TART</u>

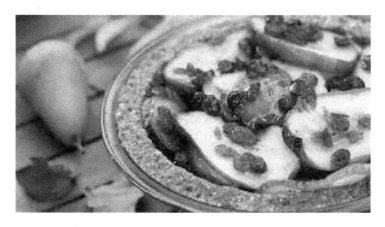

INGREDIENTS

Crust

51. 2½ cups walnuts or pecans, toasted for 8 minutes in a 350° oven

52. 1 cup Medjool dates, pitted

53. ½ teaspoon cinnamon

54. sea salt to taste

Filling

55. 3 ripe pears, thinly sliced

56. ¼ teaspoon cinnamon

57. ¼ teaspoon nutmeg

58. ½ cup maple syrup

59. ¼ cup apple cider

60. ¼ cup dried cranberries

INSTRUCTIONS

61. For the Crust: Combine the walnuts, dates, cinnamon and salt in the bowl of a food processor and process until the mixture is well combined but not completely smooth. Press it into the bottom and up the sides of a nine-inch non-stick tart pan and refrigerate while you make the filling.

62. For the Filling: Place the pears, cinnamon, nutmeg, maple syrup, apple cider, and dried cranberries in a saucepan and cook over medium heat until the pears are tender, about 10 minutes. Remove the pears and cranberries with a slotted spoon to a bowl and set aside. Return the pan to the heat and cook the remaining liquid in the pan until it is reduced by half.

63. Spread the fruit over the tart crust and pour the reduced liquid over it.

64. Refrigerate until ready to serve.

45. **INDIAN BROWN RICE PUDDING (KHEER)**

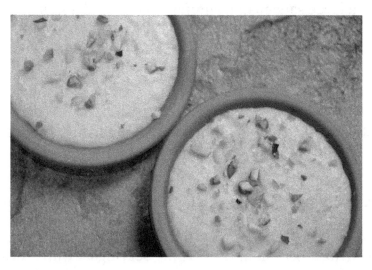

INGREDIENTS

65. 3 cups unsweetened, unflavored plant milk, such as almond, soy, cashew, or rice

66. 1 cup dry brown rice

67. ¼ cup chopped dates

68. ¼ cup pure cane sugar or pure maple syrup

69. 2 pinches saffron

70. 1 tablespoon raisins

71. 1 tablespoon slivered or sliced almonds, toasted

72. 1 tablespoon roasted pistachios, chopped

73. 1 teaspoon ground cardamom

74. Garnishes: few strands saffron, slivered or sliced toasted almonds, chopped roasted pistachios

INSTRUCTIONS

75. In a large saucepan combine milk, rice, dates, sugar, and 1 cup water. Bring to boiling; reduce heat to low. Simmer, uncovered, about 45 minutes or until rice is completely cooked, stirring frequently. (The liquid should not be completely cooked off.)

76. Meanwhile, in a small bowl combine saffron and 3 to 4 Tbsp. hot water. Let stand 10 to 15 minutes.

77. Add saffron with soaking liquid, raisins, almonds, pistachios, cardamom, and ½ cup water to cooked rice. Cook 10 to 20 minutes more or until rice is creamy, stirring occasionally. Top servings with desired garnishes.

46. <u>SOUTHERN-STYLE BANANA PUDDING PARFAITS</u>

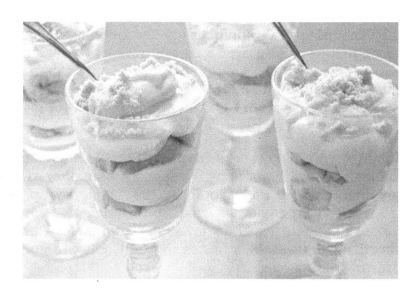

INGREDIENTS

78. ¼ cup cornstarch

79. 2 cups unsweetened, unflavored plant milk, such as almond, soy, cashew, or rice

80. 4 tablespoons + 2 teaspoons pure maple syrup

81. ⅛ teaspoon ground nutmeg

82. ⅛ teaspoon sea salt

83. 1¾ teaspoons pure vanilla extract

84. ¾ cup rolled oats

85. ¼ teaspoon ground cinnamon

86. ½ cup raw cashews, soaked overnight

87. 3 large or 4 small bananas, sliced into ¼-inch-thick rounds

INSTRUCTIONS

88. For pudding, place cornstarch in a medium saucepan. Gradually whisk in milk until smooth. Whisk in 3 tablespoons of the maple syrup, the nutmeg, and salt. Bring just to boiling over medium, whisking constantly. Cook and whisk 2 to 3 minutes more or until mixture is thickened and no foam remains on the surface. Stir in 1 teaspoon of the vanilla. Transfer to a bowl to cool.

89. While pudding cools, preheat oven to 350°F. Line a small baking sheet with parchment paper. In a small bowl stir together oats, 1 tablespoon of the maple syrup, ½ teaspoon of the vanilla, and the cinnamon. Spread mixture in a ½-inch-thick layer on the prepared baking sheet. Bake 15 to 18 minutes or until oats are golden brown, stirring once.

90. For cashew cream topping, drain cashews. In a blender combine cashews and the remaining 2 teaspoons maple syrup and ¼ teaspoon vanilla. Add ¼ cup water. Cover and blend until smooth and creamy. Place in an airtight container; chill.

91. To assemble parfaits, spoon 2 Tbsp. pudding in each of four parfait glasses. Top with one-third of the banana slices and one-third of the oat mixture. Repeat with another layer of pudding, one-third of the banana slices. and one-third of the oat mixture. Layer with the remaining banana slices and pudding. Cover and chill parfaits 1 to 8 hours.

92. Just before serving, if desired, top with additional banana slices and the remaining oat mixture. Top each with 1 tablespoon cashew cream and additional cinnamon.

47. **PURPLE STICKY RICE PUDDING**

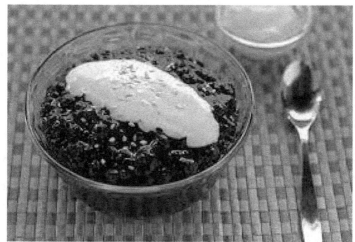

INGREDIENTS

93. ¾ cup sweet purple sticky rice

94. 1½ cups unsweetened, unflavored plant milk, such as almond, soy, cashew, or rice

95. 1 ripe banana, coarsely chopped

96. 1 vanilla bean pod, split and seeds scraped, or 1 Tbsp. pure vanilla extract

97. 1 kiwifruit, halved and sliced

98. ½ cup sliced fresh mango, kumquats, or pineapple

INSTRUCTIONS

99. In a medium saucepan combine rice, milk, banana, vanilla pod and seeds, and 1½ cups water. Bring to boiling; reduce heat. Cover and simmer about 25 minutes or until rice is tender. Remove lid; cook 1 minute more to "tighten" rice into a creamy pudding. Remove vanilla pod.

100. Serve pudding warm, chilled, or at room temperature. Top with fruit.

48. STRAWBERRY CLAFOUTI DESSERT

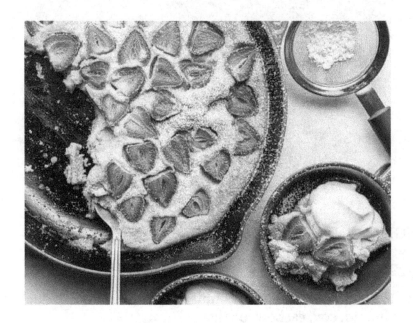

INGREDIENTS

101. 1 lb. fresh strawberries, trimmed and sliced

102. 1 lb. ripe bananas (about 3), peeled and sliced

103. 1 10-oz. jar no-sugar-added strawberry jam

104. 2 cups gluten-free rolled oats

105. 1 teaspoon regular or sodium-free baking powder

106. 1 cup unsweetened, unflavored plant-based milk

107. ½ cup unsweetened applesauce

INSTRUCTIONS

108. Preheat oven to 350°F. In a large bowl gently stir together strawberries, bananas, and jam. Transfer fruit mixture to an 8-inch square silicone baking pan.

109. In another bowl stir together oats and baking powder. Add milk and applesauce; stir to mix. Sprinkle oat mixture evenly over fruit mixture. Bake about 45 minutes or until golden brown.

49. <u>FRUIT-TOPPED VANILLA CUPCAKES</u>

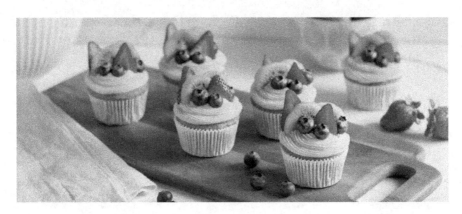

INGREDIENTS

CUPCAKES

110. ¾ cup unsweetened, unflavored plant-based milk

111. ¾ cup pure maple syrup

112. ¼ cup pure vanilla extract

113. 1 tablespoon apple cider vinegar

114. 1 tablespoon ground flaxseed

115. 1 cup oat flour

116. ¾ cup sorghum flour

117. ½ cup almond flour

118. 1 teaspoon baking powder

119. 1 teaspoon baking soda

120.   ¼ teaspoon sea salt

FROSTING AND GARNISH

121. ¾ pounds white sweet potatoes, peeled and cut into large pieces

122. ¼ cup pure maple syrup

123. 1 tablespoon tahini

124. 1 tablespoon pure vanilla extract

125. 2 kiwis, cut into half-moon slices

126. 4 small strawberries, halved

127. ¼ cup blueberries

INSTRUCTIONS

128. Preheat the oven to 335°F. Line a 12-cup muffin tin with 12 paper liners.

129. In a mixing bowl, combine milk, maple syrup, vanilla, vinegar, and flaxseed.

130. In a separate bowl whisk together the flours, baking powder, baking soda, and salt.

131. Add the wet mix to the flour and mix well.

132. Evenly divide the batter between 12 cupcake molds.

133. Bake 30 to 35 minutes or until a toothpick inserted in the center of a cupcake comes out dry.

134. Transfer cupcakes to a cooling rack and let cool completely.

135. For frosting, place yam pieces in a steamer basket in a saucepan. Add water to saucepan to just below basket.

Cover pan and steam sweet potato 20 minutes, or until very tender. Let sweet potato cool; then transfer to a food processor. Add maple syrup, tahini, and vanilla. Process until smooth and creamy.

136.   Transfer frosting to a piping bag, and pipe onto the tops of cooled cupcakes.

137.   Chill cupcakes in the fridge for an hour or until ready to serve.

138.   Just before serving, decorate tops of cupcakes with fresh fruits.

50. SWEET POTATO BITES

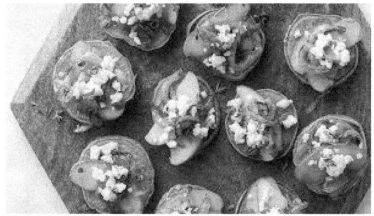

INGREDIENTS

139. 1 pound (about 3) white, orange, or purple sweet potatoes, peeled and cut into cubes

140. 1 tablespoon brown sugar

141. ⅓ cup ground peanuts, macadamia nuts, or sesame seeds

142. Dash of cinnamon

INSTRUCTIONS

143. Boil or steam the potatoes until tender, then mash potatoes with sugar.

144. Once cool enough to handle, roll potatoes into walnut-size balls.

145. On a clean surface, spread a layer of ground nuts of your choice or sesame seeds. Gently roll the potato balls in the nuts to coat.

146. Powder with cinnamon to serve.

51. CANTALOUPE-CUCUMBER SOUP

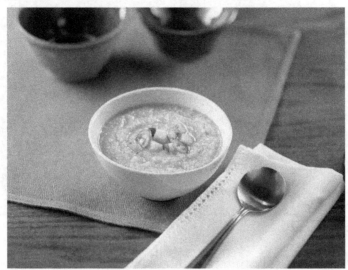

INGREDIENTS

147. 6 cups 1-inch pieces cantaloupe

148. ½ cup unsweetened almond or rice milk

149. 2 tablespoons lime juice

150. ½ teaspoon grated fresh ginger

151. ½ cup chopped, peeled, and seeded cucumber

152. Sea salt, to taste

153. 2 tablespoons finely snipped fresh basil

INSTRUCTIONS

154. In a blender combine cantaloupe, almond milk, lime juice, and ginger. Cover and blend until smooth. Add cucumber; cover and blend until smooth. Season with salt. Stir in basil. Cover and chill at least 2 hours (up to 5 hours).

155. Top servings with additional cucumber and basil.

52. <u>CHOCOLATE PISTACHIO MINT AND STRAWBERRY ROSE BLISS BALLS</u>

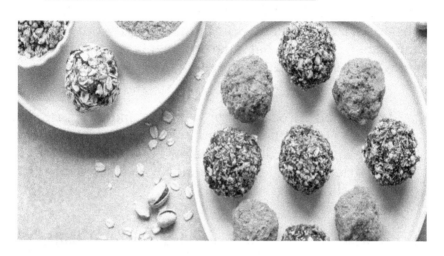

INGREDIENTS

156. 2 cups rolled oats

157. ¼ cup toasted shelled pistachios

158. ½ cup freeze-dried strawberries

159. 1 cup <u>Date Paste,</u> divided

160. ½ cup raisins, divided

161. 3 tablespoons cocoa powder

162. ½ teaspoon pure vanilla extract

163. 1 drop peppermint extract

164. 2 pinches salt, divided

165. 1 teaspoon rose water

INSTRUCTIONS

166. Combine the oats for both flavors and transfer to a warm skillet. Roast for 5 to 10 minutes on medium-low heat, stirring frequently, until the oats give out a toasted aroma. Divide the oat mixture evenly into two mixing bowls; let cool for 10 minutes.

167. In a food processor or spice grinder, pulse the pistachios to a crumbly or coarse powdery texture. Remove and set aside in a shallow bowl. Repeat with the freeze-dried strawberries. Remove and set aside in a separate shallow bowl.

168. To assemble the Chocolate Pistachio Mint Balls: Add ½ cup Date Paste, ¼ cup raisins, the cocoa powder, vanilla and peppermint extracts, and 1 pinch salt to one of the bowls of oats. Mix well. Scoop up 1 tablespoon of the mixture and roll it into a ball. Roll the chocolate ball in the crushed pistachios until coated, and set aside. Repeat until you have 16 balls.

169. To assemble the Strawberry Rose Balls, add ½ cup Date Paste, ¼ cup raisins, the rose water, and 1 pinch salt to the remaining bowl of oats. Mix well. Scoop up 1 tablespoon of the mixture and roll it into a ball. Roll the ball in the crushed freeze-dried strawberries until coated. Repeat this process until you have 13 balls.

170. Store in an airtight container in the fridge until ready to serve.

53. __BROWNIES__

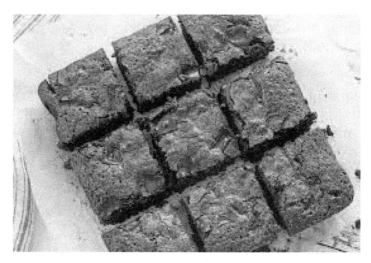

INGREDIENTS

171. 1 (15-ounce) can no-salt-added black beans, drained and rinsed (or 1½ cups cooked)

172. 1 cup pure date syrup

173. ½ cup unsweetened cocoa powder

174. ¾ cup rolled oats

175. 1 teaspoon baking powder

176. ½ teaspoon baking soda

177. Unsalted pistachio nuts, finely chopped (optional)

178. Vegan semisweet chocolate pieces (optional)

INSTRUCTIONS

179. Preheat the oven to 350°F. Line an 8- or 9-inch round cake pan with parchment paper (or use a silicone cake pan).

180. Combine the beans, date syrup, and cocoa powder in a food processor; process just until smooth. Add the oats, baking powder, and baking soda; process just until combined.

181. Spread batter into the prepared cake pan. Sprinkle with pistachios and chocolate pieces (if using). Bake for 35 minutes. Cool on a wire rack. Cut into wedges.

54. HIDDEN BERRY DESSERT SQUARES

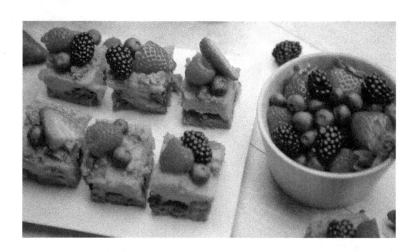

INGREDIENTS

CRUMBLE

182. 2 cups dates or date paste

183. 1½ cups whole grain bread crumbs

184. 2 teaspoons pure vanilla extract

185. 2 pinches sea salt

CREAM LAYER

186. 2 pounds unpeeled sweet potatoes, baked until tender (about 3 cups mashed)

187. 3–4 tablespoons pure cane sugar

188. 1½ tablespoons lemon zest

189. 1 tablespoon pure vanilla extract

190. 2 cups mixed fresh berries, plus more for garnish

INSTRUCTIONS

191.   Place the dates in the bowl of a food processor, and pulse to break into small bits. Add the bread crumbs, vanilla, and salt, and pulse to the texture of coarse sand.

192.   Reserve ¼ cup of the crumble for topping, and press the rest of it into the bottom of an 8-inch square baking dish. Press down to make an even, compact base layer. Transfer dish to refrigerator to chill for 20 to 30 minutes.

193.   Scoop the interior of the sweet potatoes into the bowl of a food processor, and discard potato skins. Add sugar, lemon zest, and vanilla to the sweet potato. Purée to a smooth, creamy texture.

194.   Remove the baking dish from the refrigerator, and spread a layer of fresh berries over the base layer. Cover the berries evenly with all of the sweet potato puree, and smooth the top with a spatula. Sprinkle the reserved crumble on top.

195.   Refrigerate for at least 30 minutes, or until ready to serve. To serve, cut into 16 squares, and garnish with fresh berries.

55. <u>CHERRY SOFT-SERVE ICE CREAM</u>

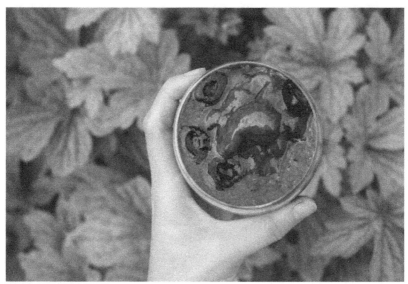

INGREDIENTS

196.   4 medium-sized bananas, cut into 1-inch pieces and frozen

197.   1 cup frozen cherries

198.   1/2 teaspoon vanilla extract

199.   1 tablespoon to 1/4 cup unsweetened almond milk, as needed

200.   2 tablespoons mini vegan chocolate chips

INSTRUCTIONS

201.   In a food processor, combine the frozen banana pieces, cherries, and vanilla extract.

202.   Process until creamy, adding almond milk one tablespoon at a time as necessary.

203.   Pulse in the chocolate chips. Serve immediately.

56. FRUIT & SPICE COOKIES

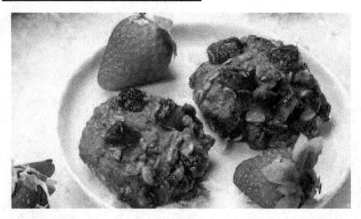

INGREDIENTS

204.   3 cups rolled oats, divided

205.   1 teaspoon ground cinnamon

206.   ½ teaspoon ground nutmeg

207.   ½ teaspoon ground cloves

208.   1 tablespoon baking powder

209.   3 tablespoons ground flaxseeds

210.   1 cup applesauce, no added sugar

211.1¼ cup strawberry fruit spread, no added sugar

212.   8 dates, pitted and diced

213.   ¾ cup pecan pieces

INSTRUCTIONS

214.   Preheat the oven to 375°F. Line two baking sheets with parchment paper. Mix 1½ cups of the rolled oats, the baking powder, and the spices (cinnamon, nutmeg, and cloves) in a large bowl and set aside.

215.   In either a blender or food processor, combine the ground flaxseed, ¾ cup water, applesauce, and the remaining 1½ cups of rolled oats. Process until the batter has an even consistency. Then, add the strawberry jam, and blend for a few seconds to combine.

216.   Pour the fruit mixture into the bowl of dry ingredients. Whisk until everything is evenly mixed. Then stir in the dates and pecans. The mixture should be slightly wet; don't expect to shape the cookies into balls.

217.   Drop 12 spoonfuls of dough onto each baking sheet. Bake for 15 to 20 minutes. Let the cookies cool for a few minutes and then enjoy warm! Store any uneaten cookies in an airtight container at room temperature for up to 2 days or in the refrigerator for up to 6 days

Recipe

_____

_____

_____

_____

_____

_____

_____

_____

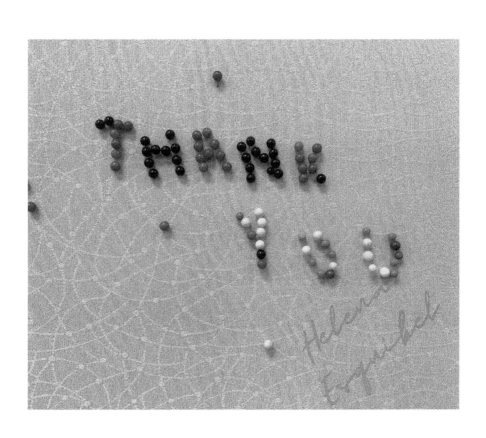

CPSIA information can be obtained
at www.ICGtesting.com
Printed in the USA
BVHW080738140521
607270BV00005B/681